D1710785

Microarray Technology and Cancer Gene Profiling

ADVANCES IN EXPERIMENTAL MEDICINE AND BIOLOGY

Recent Volumes in this Series

A Continuation Order Plan is available for this series. A continuation order will bring delivery of each new volume immediately upon publication. Volumes are billed only upon actual shipment. For further information please contact the publisher.

Microarray Technology
and Cancer Gene Profiling

Edited by

Simone Mocellin, M.D., Ph.D.

*Clinica Chirurgica II, Dipartimento di Scienze Oncologiche e Chirurgiche,
  University of Padova, Padova, Italy*

Springer Science+Business Media, LLC
Landes Bioscience / Eurekah.com

Springer Science+Business Media, LLC
Landes Bioscience / Eurekah.com

Printed in the U.S.A.

Springer Science+Business Media, LLC, 233 Spring Street, New York, New York 10013, U.S.A.
http://www.springer.com

Please address all inquiries to the Publishers:
Landes Bioscience / Eurekah.com, 1002 West Avenue, Second Floor, Austin, Texas 78701, U.S.A.
Phone: 512/ 637 6050; FAX: 512/ 637 6079
http://www.eurekah.com
http://www.landesbioscience.com

Microarray Technology and Cancer Gene Profiling, edited by Simone Mocellin, Landes Bioscience /
Springer Science+Business Media, LLC dual imprint / Springer Science+Business Media, LLC series:
Advances in Experimental Medicine and Biology

ISBN: 0-387-39977-1

While the authors, editors and publisher believe that drug selection and dosage and the specifications
and usage of equipment and devices, as set forth in this book, are in accord with current recommendations and practice at the time of publication, they make no warranty, expressed or implied, with
respect to material described in this book. In view of the ongoing research, equipment development,
changes in governmental regulations and the rapid accumulation of information relating to the biomedical
sciences, the reader is urged to carefully review and evaluate the information provided herein.

Library of Congress Cataloging-in-Publication Data

Microarray technology and cancer gene profiling / edited by Simone
   Mocellin.
      p. ; cm. -- (Advances in experimental medicine and biology ; v.
593)
   Includes bibliographical references and index.
   ISBN 0-387-39977-1
   1. Oncogenes. 2. DNA microarrays.   I. Mocellin, Simone.
   II. Series.
   [DNLM: 1. Neoplasms--genetics. 2. Gene Expression Profiling
--methods. 3. Microarray Analysis--methods.   W1 AD559 v.593
2006 / QZ 200 M626 2006]
   RC268.42.M53 2006
   616.99'4042--dc22

                              2006026465

DEDICATION

To my family

INTRODUCTION

Cancer is a heterogeneous disease in most respects, including its cellularity, different genetic alterations and diverse clinical behaviors. The combinatorial origin, the heterogeneity of malignant cells, and the variable host background produce multiple tumor subclasses. Many analytical methods have been used to study human tumors and to classify them into homogeneous groups that can predict clinical behavior. Currently, cancer classifications are principally based on clinical and histomorphologic features that only partially reflect this heterogeneity, reducing the probability of the most appropriate diagnostic, prognostic and therapeutic strategy for each patient. Furthermore, virtually all current anticancer agents do not differentiate between cancerous and normal cells, resulting in sometimes disastrous toxicity and an inconstant efficacy. The development of innovative drugs that selectively target cancer cells while sparing normal tissues is very promising and underscores the importance of dissecting the cascade of molecular events that underlie cancer development, progression and sensitivity to antineoplastic agents. Since these phenomena are sustained by the derangement of multiple genes, biotechnological tools allowing the simultaneous study of hundreds or thousands of molecular targets are greatly welcome and provide investigators with a unique opportunity to decipher the many enigmas that surround cell physiology and disease. Over the last decade—prompted also by the sequencing of the human genome—investigators have devised several gene expression profiling methods, such as comparative genomic hybridization (CGH), differential display, serial analysis of gene expression (SAGE), and DNA arrays. The availability of such large amounts of information has shifted the attention of scientists towards a non-reductionist approach to biological phenomena. High throughput technologies can be used to follow changing patterns of gene expression over time. Among them, DNA arrays have become prominent because they are easier to use, do not require large-scale DNA sequencing, and allow the parallel quantification of thousands of genes from multiple samples. Hopefully, by integrating this powerful analytic tool with other high throughput techniques, such as tissue microarray and proteomics, investigators will be able to comprehensively describe the molecular portrait of the biological phenomena underlying tumor pathogenesis, aggressiveness and response to therapy.

DNA array technology is rapidly spreading worldwide and has the potential to drastically change the therapeutic approach to patients affected with tumor: accordingly, it is of paramount importance for both researchers and clinicians to know the principles underlying this laboratory tool in order to critically appreciate the results originating from this biotechnology.

In the present book, we describe the main features of microarray technology—from DNA array construction to data analysis—and discuss its key applications by reviewing some of the most interesting results already achieved in the field of oncology.

Simone Mocellin, M.D., Ph.D.

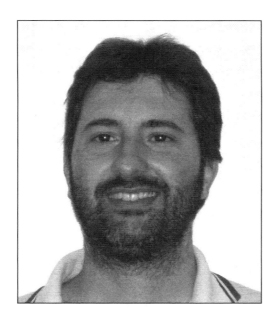

ABOUT THE EDITOR...

SIMONE MOCELLIN, M.D., Ph.D. graduated in Medicine at the Medical School of the University of Padova, Italy, where he received his Ph.D. in the antineoplastic activity of tumor necrosis factor (TNF). He spent two years at the Surgery Branch, National Cancer Institute, NIH, Bethesda, Maryland, U.S.A., where he was involved in translational and clinical research in the field of oncology. Currently, he is a clinical attendant at the Surgery Branch, Department of Oncological and Surgical Sciences, University of Padova, Italy. His main research interests include innovative approaches for the treatment of solid malignancies (e.g., melanoma, soft tissue sarcomas, gastrointestinal carcinomas), such as TNF-based locoregional therapies and molecularly targeted antineoplastic strategies (e.g., cancer vaccines, identification of minimal residual disease and tumor molecular profiling for optimization of cancer treatment).

x

PARTICIPANTS

Giovanni Esposito
Department of Oncological
  and Surgical Sciences
University of Padova
Padova
Italy

Marianna Fantin
Pharmacology Section
Department of Pharmacology
  and Anesthesiology
University of Padova
Padova
Italy

Elena M. Hartmann
Institute of Pathology
University of Würzburg
Würzburg
Germany

Mei He
Surgery Branch
National Cancer Institute
National Institutes of Health
Bethesda, Maryland
U.S.A.

Sarah E. Henrickson
Institute of Pathology
University of Würzburg
Würzburg
Germany

Ernest S. Kawasaki
SAIC-Frederick, Inc.
National Cancer Institute
Gaithersburg, Maryland
U.S.A.

Ming Lei
Pel-Freez Biologicals
Rogers, Arkansas
U.S.A.

Steven K. Libutti
Surgery Branch
National Cancer Institute
National Institutes of Health
Bethesda, Maryland
U.S.A.

Mario Lise
Clinica Chirurgica II
Dipartimento di Scienze Oncologiche
  e Chirurgiche
University of Padova
Padova, Italy

Robert Luhm
Pel-Freez Biologicals
Rogers, Arkansas
U.S.A.

Susanna Mandruzzato
Oncology Section
Department of Oncological
    and Surgical Sciences
University of Padova
Padova
Italy

David Mangiameli
Surgery Branch
National Cancer Institute
National Institutes of Health
Bethesda, Maryland
U.S.A.

Francesco M. Marincola
Department of Transfusion Medicine
Immunogenetics Section
National Institutes of Health
Bethesda, Maryland
U.S.A.

Simone Mocellin
Clinica Chirurgica II
Dipartimento di Scienze Oncologiche
    e Chirurgiche
University of Padova
Padova
Italy

Vladia Monsurrò
Department of Transfusion Medicine
Immunogenetics Section
National Institutes of Health
Bethesda, Maryland
U.S.A.

Andrey Morgun
Ghost Lab
Laboratory of Cellular
    and Molecular Immunology
NIAID
National Institutes of Health
Bethesda, Maryland
U.S.A.

Donato Nitti
Clinica Chirurgica II
Dipartimento di Scienze Oncologiche
    e Chirurgiche
University of Padova
Padova
Italy

Lucy O'Donovan
Yoshitomi Research Institute
    of Neuroscience (YRING)
University of Glasgow
Glasgow
U.K.

German Ott
Institute of Pathology
University of Würzburg
Würzburg
Germany

Monica Panelli
Immunogenetics Section
Department of Transfusion Medicine
Clinical Center
National Institutes of Health
Bethesda, Maryland
U.S.A.

Ainhoa Perez-Diez
Ghost Lab
Laboratory of Cellular
   and Molecular Immunology
NIAID
National Institutes of Health
Bethesda, Maryland
U.S.A.

David W. Petersen
SAIC-Frederick, Inc.
National Cancer Institute
Gaithersburg, Maryland
U.S.A.

Maurizio Provenzano
Clinica Chirurgica II
Dipartimento di Scienze Oncologiche
   e Chirurgiche
University of Padova
Padova
Italy

Vilda Purutcuoglu
Department of Mathematics
   and Statistics
Lancaster University
Lancaster
U.K.

Luigi Quintieri
Pharmacology Section
Department of Pharmacology
   and Anesthesiology
University of Padova
Padova
Italy

Jennifer Rosen
Surgery Branch
National Cancer Institute
National Institutes of Health
Bethesda, Maryland
U.S.A.

Andreas Rosenwald
Institute of Pathology
University of Würzburg
Würzburg
Germany

Carlo Riccardo Rossi
Clinica Chirurgica II
Dipartimento di Scienze Oncologiche
   e Chirurgiche
University of Padova
Padova
Italy

Natalia Shulzhenko
Ghost Lab
Laboratory of Cellular
   and Molecular Immunology
NIAID
National Institutes of Health
Bethesda, Maryland
U.S.A.

Csaba Vizler
Pharmacology Section
Department of Pharmacology
   and Anesthesiology
University of Padova
Padova
Italy

Ena Wang
Immunogenetics Section
Department of Transfusion Medicine
Clinical Center
National Institutes of Health
Bethesda, Maryland
U.S.A.

Lu Wang
Pel-Freez Biologicals
Rogers, Arkansas
U.S.A.

Ernst Wit
Medical Statistics Unit
Department of Mathematics
  and Statistics
Lancaster University
Lancaster
U.K.

Ximin Zhu
Department of Mathematics
  and Statistics
Lancaster University
Lancaster
U.K.

CONTENTS

SECTION II: APPLICATIONS IN THE ONCOLOGY FIELD

10. CANCER DEVELOPMENT AND PROGRESSION 117

Mei He, Jennifer Rosen, David Mangiameli and Steven K. Libutti

11. GENE EXPRESSION PROFILING IN MALIGNANT
LYMPHOMAS 134

Sarah E. Henrickson, Elena M. Hartmann, German Ott
    and Andreas Rosenwald

12. TUMOR IMMUNOLOGY 147

Simone Mocellin, Mario Lise and Donato Nitti

CHAPTER 1

Manufacturing of Microarrays

David W. Petersen* and Ernest S. Kawasaki

Abstract

DNA microarray technology has become a powerful tool in the arsenal of the molecular biologist. Capitalizing on high precision robotics and the wealth of DNA sequences annotated from the genomes of a large number of organisms, the manufacture of microarrays is now possible for the average academic laboratory with the funds and motivation. Microarray production requires attention to both biological and physical resources, including DNA libraries, robotics, and qualified personnel. While the fabrication of microarrays is a very labor-intensive process, production of quality microarrays individually tailored on a project-by-project basis will help researchers shed light on future scientific questions.

Introduction

In the past ten years the use of microarrays has gone from a cutting edge novelty to a well-defined technique in most molecular biology laboratories. With the availability of affordable, high precision robotics, the production of high-density microarrays is accessible to anyone with the determination, will and funding. Ever since Patrick Brown's laboratory at Stanford University popularized the method, the allure to print one's own microarrays has been enticing.[1,2] And why not? The basic concept of printing microarrays is exceedingly simple. Very small spots of DNA solutions of different DNA species are placed on a slide several thousand times. However, looks can be deceiving. Manufacturing microarrays is a very labor-intensive process, even with the use of robotics, and obtaining meaningful and useful results can still be as difficult as ever. This chapter will provide a brief overview of the manufacturing of microarrays in an academic setting. It is not intended as a detailed instruction manual, but rather an overview of the process that highlights the critical decisions needed to manufacture one's own microarrays. To successfully embark on the mission of manufacturing microarrays will require more information than this text can provide, but by the end of this chapter, one should understand the major elements of production and resource allocation needed to make a high-quality microarray.

Nomenclature

While the term "microarray" is used to describe a variety of devices, for these purposes a microarray is a miniaturized, ordered arrangement of nucleic acid fragments located at defined positions on a solid support, enabling the analysis of thousands of genes in parallel. This discussion will be confined to the manufacture of mRNA expression microarrays. While many more devices are also called microarrays, we will leave the details of producing BAC arrays,

*Corresponding Author: David W. Petersen—SAIC-Frederick, Inc., National Cancer Institute, Microarray Facility 8717 Grovemont Circle, Rm. 128; Gaithersburg, Maryland, U.S.A. Email: petersed@mail.nih.gov

Microarray Technology and Cancer Gene Profiling, edited by Simone Mocellin.
©2007 Landes Bioscience and Springer Science+Business Media.

protein arrays, tissue arrays, etc. for other publications. However, once one becomes adept at printing DNA microarrays, those skills will prove invaluable in other microarraying endeavors.

To clarify nomenclature, the spots, or elements, on the array are printed from a DNA library. This DNA library contains the known sequences, and so the printed features should be referred to as the probe. The unknown sequence is from the labeled target RNA sample. The instrument that prints microarrays can be referred to as a gridder, printer, printing robot, microarraying robot, etc.

The DNA Microarray Library

The most important aspect of building a microarray, which often becomes overshadowed by the technological hardware issues, is the DNA library.

In the beginning, microarrays were manufactured with cDNA assembled from available clone libraries. Generally these libraries were gathered as part of larger genomic sequencing efforts and then made available to groups printing microarrays. Typically the DNA was cloned in bacterial vectors with universal primers that allowed PCR amplification of the libraries in order to generate high concentration of pure DNA that corresponded to an expressed gene.

Today, research groups are increasingly switching to presynthesized, long oligonucleotide libraries as the printing libraries of choice. As of this writing, the field of companies supplying large oligonucleotide expression libraries has been winnowed down to Operon and Illumina. Libraries from both of these companies work well, so the decision of their use should be made based on available genomic content. These companies are continually improving the libraries as more genomic information becomes annotated. As the genomic sequence information becomes more complete, oligos can be designed for any known gene for sequenced organisms. Oligonucleotides of 60-70 bases in length show the best sensitivity and specificity.[3,4] Moreover oligonucleotide libraries are easier to maintain. Because they can always be resynthesized they can be digitally archived in a computer database, so there is no need to keep a permanent physical copy in a -80°C freezer. Use of oligonucleotide libraries also eliminates the possibility of cross-contamination during PCR or bacterial propagation. As human error cannot be eliminated, cross-contamination of oligo libraries might occur by well-to-well splashing caused by careless handling.

One detail of microarray DNA libraries of any type that is often overlooked is the care and maintenance of the plate sets. For any library of significant size (>10,000 features), it is highly advisable to have access to a liquid handling system for microwell plates. While printing from 96-well plates is possible, 384-well microtiter plates are required for an array to be printed with reasonable speed. If your facility is committed to constructing a PCR-amplified cDNA array, you will probably begin with clones in 96-well microtiter plates. Access to many thermal cyclers (≥ eight 96-well cyclers) is needed for a moderate throughput of samples so that the library can be completed in a timely manner. At some point in the process one will have to transfer four 96-well plates into one 384-well plate. In order to accomplish this without error, a liquid handling robot with a 96 pipette-tip head is recommended. As the need for high-throughput systems has increased, the market has responded and a large variety of liquid handling systems are now available. Speed and flexibility of the liquid handler are the primary concerns, followed closely by reliability and quality service. Presynthesized oligonucleotide libraries are available already aliquoted in 384-well microtiter plates. While a 96-pipette tip head will suffice, a 384-tip robot will greatly increase the speed of any subsequent handling of the library.

Careful thought and foresight should also be used when determining the printing buffer in which to resuspend the library. This topic will be covered more fully in the section on substrate selection, but keep in mind that once the library is resuspended in a buffer, it will be virtually impossible to change. The buffer chosen will determine the optimal storage and handling of the library and each choice has its own merits. Most importantly, the DNA library needs to be resuspended at the proper concentration before printing. For cDNA probes the concentration should range between 100-500 ng/μl. As cDNA libraries typically contain PCR products sized from 200 to 2000bp, the concentration and viscosity can vary from well to well. The most common mistake that groups make when they prepare cDNA libraries for microarraying is that the final DNA concentration per well is simply too low. Whether they are trying to save money by using less thermostable polymerase (i.e., Taq) or if the DNA becomes lost during purification, the consequence of DNA amounts that are too dilute is a poor array. Spot shape is highly dependent on the DNA concentration, and doughnut-shaped and crescent-shaped spots are almost always caused by insufficient concentration of DNA.

Oligo libraries come from the manufacturer in aliquots that should already be normalized by mass. One can follow the recommended printing concentrations from the manufacturers. We have found 20 μM to be the low end of the concentration range, and 40 μM should be in vast excess. Some well-to-well variability in the oligo concentrations exists, but using a dilution between 25-30 μM works quite well. Oligo libraries are easier to print than the cDNA libraries in general, because oligos are more even in concentration and viscosity.

The final consideration with DNA libraries is having a good computerized record keeping/ database system in place. Before a single DNA spot is printed, make sure that all of relevant sequence and gene information will be available. In particular this can cause frustration when comparing different libraries, especially if one library uses UniGene identifiers and another uses Refseq or Ensemble, and a common identifier is not in the original information. As the sizes of available libraries keep increasing, the bioinformatics can become an issue if one is not adequately prepared.

Robotic Printers

A printing robot needs to have motion control in three axes with an accuracy of +/- 5 μm (Fig. 1). The better the accuracy of the printer, the more features can be printed in a single array. There are two approaches to obtaining a printing robot: self-assembly or commercial purchase.

Self-assembly of a printing robot requires access to talented individuals with abilities in both electronics and engineering. A university engineering department might be a good place to ask for assistance. Probably the most common 'home-built" arrayer is based on the designs that have been made publicly available by the Brown Lab at Stanford University. The "M-Guide" (http://cmgm.stanford.edu/pbrown/mguide/index.html) has instructions for building one's own arrayer, an endeavor not recommended for those who are unable to invest a lot of "sweat equity" or for those who want quick results.

For those who are less inclined towards engineering, several printing robots are available commercially, though they all have their strengths and weaknesses. From a purely statistical viewpoint one would expect that the more moving parts a machine has, the more likely that one of those parts will fail. But experience shows that the quality of the components and the care in construction and engineering are often a better predictor of reliability. Before making a major purchase it is strongly advisable to talk to researchers who are actually using the printer under consideration and get their honest opinion of how well it operates. While reliability is primarily important, ease of use and the software capabilities should also influence the decision. Some printing robots can only be calibrated by the company technician, while others allow the user complete access to the machine calibration. A very important factor outside of the basic engineering concerns is how much customer support does the company provide?

For either approach, the first consideration should be the desired through-put of the arrayer. Arrayers are available that will print 25, 50, 100 or > 200 slides in a print run. If fewer than 50 arrays at a time are needed, a smaller instrument may be sufficient. Keep in mind that a high through-put machine can always be used to print a smaller number of arrays than the full capacity.

A second critical criterion of any arrayer is the pin-washing station. In order to limit or eliminate potential carryover, the washing station must be able to thoroughly remove all of the DNA from one sample before picking up the next one. In addition, failure to completely clean and dry the pins before the next sampling could lead to carryover and/or pin failure.

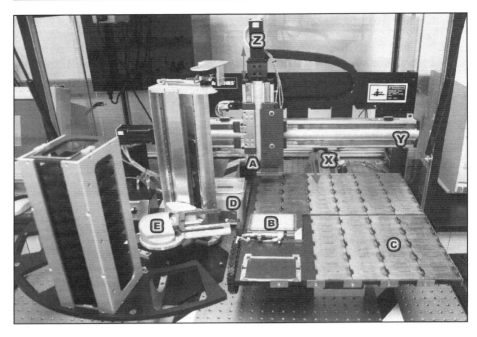

Figure 1. The major components of a microarray printer: X, Y and Z) axis motion controllers. A) Print head, moves in the Y and Z axis. B) Plate nest, holds sample plate. C) Slide holders, immobilizes the array on the printing platter, which moves in the X axis. D) Wash station. E) Automated plate handler.

Finally, regardless of the printing arrayer used, the calibration of the robot is absolutely critical. The tolerances needed are very tight, and every micron out of "true" can cause problems. Quite often what may seem to be a printing failure is in reality caused by poor calibration. For example, an initial observation of pins that do not print in fact may be due to incorrect position of the pins in the drying station so that the pins do not dry properly. Additionally, improper calibration of plate position may cause the robot to move precisely to the incorrect position.

It should be mentioned at this point that the choice of microtiter plate type that will hold your printing library is not trivial. Most importantly it will have to be compatible with the printing robot that one intends to use. For example, if the robot has an automatic plate handler, the plate must be the appropriate dimensions and stiffness for proper functioning. Even though there are industry standards for microtiter plate dimensions, not all manufacturers can make plates to the same tolerances, particularly if the centers of the well-to-well distances are expected to be +/-2 microns. If printing with 16 pins the variation may not be as apparent as with 48 pins (Fig. 2). Most likely these plates will be printed from multiple times, so they need to be of high quality in both materials and precision.

Most commercially available robots are provided with an enclosure that will provide HEPA filtered humidified air. This is essential so that the printing process can be done in a dust-free, humidity controlled environment. Unfortunately very few robots come equipped with a dehumidifier, so if one is working in a very humid environment and the humidity needs to be lowered, the room where the robot is located may need to be dehumidified. Ideally, the building where the robot is located will have conditioned air that will keep the temperature and humidity in a "good" range, typically around 25°C, 50% humidity.

Additionally, the optimal location for the printing robot is a dust-free environment; preferably the entire room should be supplied with HEPA filtered air. Even if the robot has a dust-free

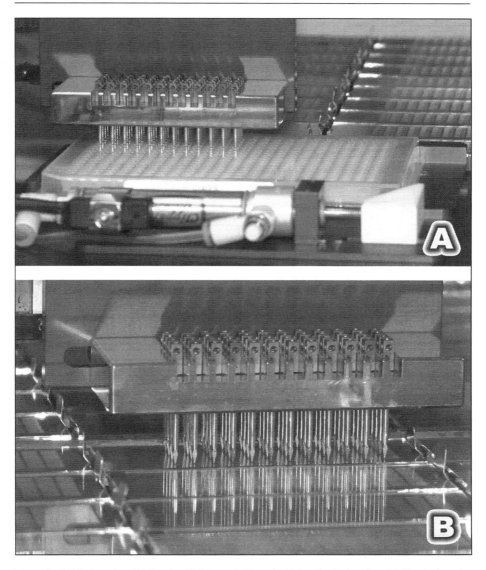

Figure 2. A) Printing pins withdrawing DNA sample from the 384 well printing plate. B) 48 printing pins spotting on the substrate.

enclosure, the slides have to be loaded by hand, with access doors allowing dust infiltration. A single piece of dirt or dust can clog a printing pin and ruin the whole print.

Printing Pins

The printing pin is the heart of the entire microarray manufacturing process. Once the robot is calibrated and the DNA library is at the proper concentration in the appropriate plates, the pins must reliably print every spot on every array.

Several types of printing pins employing different technologies are available. These include the ring-and-pin system; piezo-electric spotters; ink-jet printers; and quill-type split pins.

The ring-and-pin system employs a ring that picks up a droplet of solution and a pin that passes through the drop to deposit the solution on the substrate. The main drawbacks to this system is that it withdraws ~1 µl of solution, and the spots are relatively large ≥ 200 µm, making this suitable only for low density arrays.

Both the piezo-electric spotters and ink-jet printers are noncontact printing systems. While these systems have many potential advantages they are typically complicated with the concomitant problems of maintenance and reliability. The ink-jet system in particular has been successfully used by Agilent Technologies to manufacture their commercially available microarray, and there are even designs available for in-house custom fabrication.[5]

Although one may want to investigate different printing technologies, the simplest, most robust method utilizes contact printing with a quill-type printing pin. The quill-type printing pin operates on the same technological principle as the quill and ink pen used for over a millennium, drawing up DNA solution instead of ink in the slot through capillary action and depositing a spot by contacting the surface of the substrate. The liquid in the pin must make contact with the substrate so that the spot will be drawn out and left behind through surface tension.

Quill-type microarraying pins can be made from different materials. The most common pin used is made from a stainless steel alloy. Even though steel is a strong metal with good compression strength, it becomes fragile and delicate when miniaturized to a ~50 µm point. As the pin repeatedly touches the slide surface there will be wear on the tip. Over time the tip may become deformed, preventing the tip from either drawing up a sample or printing a spot. To address this deficiency alternative materials have been employed, notably tungsten and silicon (Fig. 3). While harder than steel, these materials are also more brittle, and silicon pins in particular are quite fragile. Whichever pin type one chooses, all pins are very small and delicate and extra care should be taken to prevent damage during handling.

The principle of capillary action that makes the quill type pin so robust and simple is also its Achilles heel. If any dirt or dust accumulates in the slot, the pin will not draw up the DNA solution. If the two tines of the pin are not perfectly even and do not touch the substrate at the same moment, the liquid may not touch the substrate and no spot will be deposited. On occasion the pin may stop printing after only printing on the first portion of the array set. This is typically caused by dirt or contaminants collecting farther up in the slot of the pin and preventing the pin from picking up a full load, or by having humidity levels too low, causing the liquid to dry out in the pin before the printing is completed.

The most common cause of a pin failure is when the pin becomes dirty or clogged. Contaminants can be picked up during the printing, and may not be sufficiently washed off. Even if the wash-dry cycle on the robot is working properly, the pins may still need to be removed from the print head and periodically given a thorough cleaning. The pin manufacturer should give recommendations for cleaning solutions and methods, often employing a sonicator. The frequency and thoroughness of pin cleaning usually is determined by personal preference, but printing pins can never be too clean.

Even using as much care as possible when setting up a print run, there will always be the possibility of a piece of dust getting in and clogging the pin. To try to determine the cause of a pin failure requires the removal of the pin and visual inspection, employing a high-quality stereo dissecting scope. While there will be times when there is no apparent cause of failure, often the problem might be noticeable, such as an offending dust particle trapped in the slot or a bent tip. If the problem is a piece of dust, it can be carefully removed. It may be (remotely) possible to repair a damaged tip with careful 'microsurgery', but the failure rate is high, and it is usually better to replace the damaged pin. As accidents can and will happen, it is a good idea to always have some extra pins available for this reason.

If the printing robot operates within proper tolerances, the amount of "wobble" the pins will exhibit during the print run will be determined by the alignment and tolerances of the pin in the print head. Most available print head / pin combinations are designed so that this is not a significant issue, but if the holes in the print head become worn, the amount of "play" will become unacceptable.

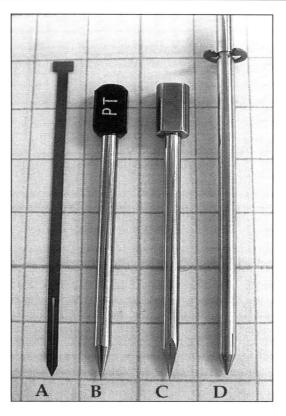

Figure 3. Four kinds of quill-type printing pins: A) Silicon. B) Tungsten. C) Stainless steel, gravity return. D) Stainless steel, spring return.

The printing parameters chosen will generally be determined by what is optimal for the printing pin (and printing buffer) in use. Typically these will need to be empirically determined once the system is installed and calibrated. The initial parameters should follow the printing pin manufacturers' recommendations. Before an actual print run with the real library and slides is attempted one should perform "test prints." In order to do test prints make a simple reagent by dissolving some DNA in the chosen printing buffer (see "slide substrates" below) and load this in the same printing plates that will be used. This will prove to be an invaluable technique to determine the expected performance of the system and to verify that all of the pins are printing properly. While some robots have a test-printing mode as a separate function, other instruments will require making a dummy run. The type of DNA used is not critical, as long as it is sheared to a small size simulating the DNA library. The concentration should be similar to the library, as spot morphology is affected by the concentration of DNA. However, an exact simulation is not necessary, and we use sheared salmon sperm DNA at a concentration of ~500 ng/µl, even though our library is composed of long oligos at ~30 µM. The point is that one needs to be sure that all of the pins draw up sufficient DNA and are printing properly and that the wash cycle is sufficient.

For printing performance the most relevant parameters are Z-axis speed, sample wicking time, dwell time, and wash cycle. A clean pin should easily wick the DNA solution in a second or less, but more viscous solutions may require longer time in the sample plate. The amount of solution in the plate will determine how far up the outside of the pin shaft the solution will go, determining pin cleaning parameters. The speed at which the pin is removed from the sample plate will also affect the amount of excess solution on the outside of the pin, which in turn determines how many of the first spots printed will be larger (which is why many groups "preblot" the pins before printing on the array slides). The Z-axis speed at which the pins touch the array slide will affect the spot size and wear on the pin. While a faster axis speed will decrease the time to print the array, it will also wear the pins down more over time. The spot size can also be controlled by the dwell time the pin touches the slide. Too long a dwell will make spots too large, and too short may mean inconsistent spotting. One of the most critical parameters is the pin wash cycle, which must wash the pins well enough to prevent cross contamination of the sample wells, and dry the pin completely so that pin wicking occurs. Each type of robot has unique wash/dry stations, and so the optimal number of wash cycles and timing parameters must be determined through trial and error.

During a test print the minimum spot-to-spot spacing achievable with the selected pin/ buffer/substrate combination should be determined. Because the test print solution is homogeneous the spots will be more uniform than the actual DNA library. So with that in mind, be aware that the densities possible during test printing will often be at least 5 μm closer together than the final microarray.

Microarray Slide Substrates

The essential choice in choosing a suitable substrate is whether to coat slides in-house or buy commercially prepared slides. Whether purchased or home-made, the same principles apply for determining a good substrate. The slide must be clean and dust free, enhance active binding of DNA to the surface, and be sufficiently hydrophobic. The more hydrophobic the slide surface is the smaller the spots will be. Smaller spots are required in order to achieve high-density arrays. While the DNA binding capacity of the substrate is clearly important, it is difficult to measure experimentally. The best indication of substrate performance is to empirically determine the signal-to-noise ratio. In general we have found that slides (and protocols) that give lower inherent background have the best signal-to-noise ratio.

Several slide coatings are in use, with the most common types being poly-L-lysine, aminosilane, and epoxy. Poly-L-lysine and aminosilane give a positive charge to the slide surface, allowing the negatively charged DNA to bind to the slide electrostatically. With epoxy coatings, the epoxy group binds covalently to DNA, especially to amino-modified oligonucleotides.

With careful selection of blank slides, a good cleaning procedure and attention to detail, "home-made" coated slides will work quite well. However, both inherent and person-to-person variability exists in any hand-coating method. Good protocols for coating slides with poly-L-lysine are available on the web at http://www.microarrays.org/ and http://derisilab.ucsf.edu/ (site maintained by the Derisi lab). Poly-L-lysine slides need to be aged >2 weeks, but should be used within 3 months. The longer the slide is aged, the more hydrophobic the surface becomes, however the background may increase if the slide is too old.

In order to minimize variability and manufacturing defects we recommend using coated slides from a reputable manufacturer. While the initial costs of buying commercially prepared coated slides seem high, the savings in successful hybridizations and fewer failed experiments pays for itself. The background from commercial slides tends to be lower and more even, giving more reliable data over the array. Most commercial slides are sent in airtight heat-sealed foil pouches. Once slide packages are opened they are subject to oxidation, and so they should be used immediately for optimal performance.

When considering the substrate to print on, one must also decide on the correct printing buffer in which to resuspend the DNA library. There are perhaps as many opinions on printing buffers as there are labs printing microarrays. Spot size and morphology are the primary considerations when choosing a substrate/buffer combination. While the print pin size determines the minimum possible spot size, the surface tension of the droplet of DNA solution on the slide substrate will determine the final spot size. The more hydrophobic the slide and the higher the surface tension, the smaller the spot will be. The same exact printing pin can print spot diameters from 75 μm to 130 μm depending on the substrate/buffer used.

As mentioned earlier, the concentration of DNA in the solution is critical. Printing with DNA at too low a concentration will leave irregular and doughnut-shaped spots. Too much DNA can make the solution too viscous, leaving bigger spots. But assuming that the DNA library is fairly well normalized, the problem of spots running together occurs when attempting to print at densities higher than the surface tension will allow. If only printing low-density arrays (spot-to-spot spacing > 250 μm) the choice of buffer and substrate will not matter in regards to spot size.

Two commonly used printing buffers are 50% DMSO and 3X SSC. The advocates of 50% DMSO like to print with it because it leaves spots with consistently round and even spot morphology. DMSO buffers are also used to reduce the evaporation rate of the solution in the printing plates. The major objection to printing with DMSO buffers is that the spots tend to be much larger than with aqueous salt buffers, and the final spot size is tremendously affected by the ambient humidity. To print a high-density array with DMSO buffer the humidity may need to be kept below 30%, which is exceedingly difficult unless one is printing in an arid environment. And if the humidity increases in the middle of a print run, the spots can start to run together.

If one lives in a region where the humidity can get quite high (as in some areas during the summer), DMSO may not be a good choice, and 3X SSC (or a similar salt buffer) may be more appropriate. The advantages of 3X SSC are that the spots stay small, and printing can be done between 50% to 65% humidity, which is usually easier to maintain.

If epoxy-coated slides are the chosen substrates, an amino-modified DNA library is preferred for optimal covalent binding. However amino-modification is not essential with long oligos or PCR products, as there are available amino-groups on the DNA polymer for binding with the epoxy-group. Optimal pH for covalent binding of the amino groups to the epoxy group is basic, between pH 8.0 to 9.0. Typically phosphate buffers (between 50 to 300mM $NaPO_4$) are used with epoxy coatings, because Tris based buffers contain amino groups that would compete for binding sites.

Commercially available printing buffers are also available, some that are specially formulated to work with the manufacturer's slide substrates. The buffers are proprietary formulations however, and one might hesitate to resuspend large and expensive DNA libraries in an unknown solution. That caveat aside, the commercial buffers should work well on the substrates for which they are designed.

Depending on the parameters to be affected, many additives may be added to printing buffers, such as betaine, ethylene glycol or detergents. 1.5M betaine can be added to the print buffer, which will reduce the evaporation rate of the spot on the slide. This will presumably increase the time for the DNA to bind to the substrate in the aqueous environment, and thereby increase amount of DNA bound to the slide.[6] Ethylene glycol reduces evaporation rates. Detergents (SDS, sarcosyl, Tween, Triton, etc.) are added to increase the spot size and improve wetting (and wicking) of the print pin. Very small amounts of detergents can make large increases in spot size, so the optimal concentration will be between 0.001% to 0.05%. The final concentration of detergent that will make the desired spot size must be empirically determined for the chosen substrate.[7] However, if the goal is to print the highest density arrays possible, avoid any extra additives, as they will lower surface tension or increase viscosity, and invariably increase the spot size (lowering the final number of features on your array).

After the array has been printed, the final step is to wash away the excess DNA and block the slide surface. If printing on homemade poly-L-lysine slides be sure to follow the "Post Processing Arrays" protocol on the DeRisi Lab page closely. This procedure uses succinic anhydride to neutralize the active amine sites on the slide and has been effectively used on commercial aminosilane slides as well. The commercial substrates will have detailed protocols in the package inserts for their recommended procedure.

Whichever method is used, the blocking step is critical to ensure low background in the final hybridization. If there is incomplete or improper blocking, all of the previous steps in the array manufacturing process will prove to have been fruitless.

Personnel

One aspect of printing microarrays that often gets overlooked in the field is attention to the people who will operate the equipment and process the arrays. Far from being an afterthought, staffing requirements are more critical than the equipment and facilities. The most expensive printing robot is useless without careful, willing, dedicated staff. As outlined above, it should be emphasized that every step is crucial, and if one part of the process goes awry, the end product is ruined. Motivated staff members who are comfortable with robotics and pay careful attention to detail are needed for an array facility to manufacture the kind of high quality arrays that yield meaningful scientific results. When selecting staff be sure to avoid careless and arrogant individuals, for they will hinder all progress in the facility.

The staff needs to maintain attention to every aspect of the process, under demanding circumstances. Mistakes are most likely to occur during the most tedious portions of the operation, and that is when vigilance is even more important. And when mistakes do happen (as they will when humans are involved) no one should feel too intimidated or embarrassed to speak up. An array facility needs to have people who take pride in their work, and who realize that good science depends on attention to detail.

Another skill necessary in the facility staff is superior problem-solving abilities. When performing quality control and analyzing the array hybridization results there are many potential causes for a failed experiment and finding solutions will often determine the success of the facility. Problems are seldom self-evident, and a thorough understanding of the entire process is needed to pinpoint the cause. Another aspect of problem solving is the humility to ask others for their opinions. The hubris to think that one has all the answers will always lead to frustration and disappointment.

Once the staff has amassed all the necessary skills, it is hoped that they will be able to become a resource to inform and teach others in the institute how to get the best results from microarrays. There is still an art to the technique of microarray hybridizations, and it needs willing and helpful teachers to be disseminated.

Conclusions

It is true that manufacturing microarrays is a very labor-intensive process, even with all of the robotic equipment to be had. However manufacturing microarrays in a research lab is easier now than ever before, thanks to the wealth of information and available resources. As more genomic information becomes annotated there will be more opportunities to mine this wealth of data, and microarrays will continue to be an invaluable tool.

For a good overview and historical perspective refer to Nature Genetics supplementary issues The Chipping Forecast (Nature Genetics 1999 January; 21(1s); The Chipping Forecast II (Nature Genetics 2002 December; 32(4s)), The Chipping Forecast III (Nature Genetics 2005 June; 37(6s).

Acknowledgements

This research was supported (in part) by the Intramural Research Program of the NIH, National Cancer Institute, Center for Cancer Research. This project has been funded in whole or in part with Federal funds from the National Cancer Institute, National Institutes of Health, under Contract No. NO1-CO-12400.

Disclaimer

The content of this publication does not necessarily reflect the views or policies of the Department of Health and Human Services, nor does mention of trade names, commercial products, or organization imply endorsement by the U.S. Government.

References

1. Schena M et al. Quantitative monitoring of gene expression patterns with a complementary DNA microarray. Science 1995; 270:467-470.
2. Schena M et al. Parallel human genome analysis: Microarray-based expression monitoring of 1000 genes. Proc Natl Acad Sci USA 1996; 93:10614-10619.
3. Hughes TR et al. Expression profiling using microarrays fabricated by an ink-jet oligonucleotide synthesizer. Nat Biotechnol 2001; 19:342-347.
4. Kane MD et al. Assessment of the sensitivity and specificity of oligonucleotide (50 mer) microarrays. Nucleic Acid Res 2000; 28:4552-4557.
5. Lausted C et al. POSaM: A fast, flexible, open-source, inkjet oligonucleotide synthesizer and microarrayer. Genome Biology 2004; 5(8):R58.
6. Diehl F et al. Manufacturing DNA microarrays of high spot homogeneity and reduced background signal. Nucl Acids Res 2001; 29(7):E38.
7. Wrobel G et al. Optimization of high-density cDNA-microarray protocols by 'design of experiments. Nucleic Acids Res 2003; 31:67.

CHAPTER 2

Technological Platforms for Microarray Gene Expression Profiling

Susanna Mandruzzato*

Abstract

By using gene microarray technology, scientists can determine in a single experiment, the expression levels of thousands of genes within a given sample. DNA microarray technology is evolving rapidly and there are now numerous high-density platforms available which differ in terms of probe content, design, deposition technology, labeling and hybridization protocols. However, two major platforms for high-density microarray manufacture are in common use. The first utilizes robotic deposition or "spotting" of DNA molecules, while the second uses short oligonucleotides synthesized in situ.

Principles of Gene Microarray Technology

Determining the level at which genes are expressed is called microarray expression analysis, and the arrays used in this kind of analysis are called "expression chips". The basic concept of this microarray analysis is the following: RNA is harvested from a sample of interest (e.g., cell lines, tissue biopsy) and labeled to generate the target, i.e., the free nucleic acid sample whose identity or abundance is to be detected. The target is then hybridized to the probe DNA sequences corresponding to specific genes that have been affixed, in a known configuration, onto a solid matrix.

Hybridization between probe and target provides a quantitative measure of the abundance of a particular sequence in the target population. This information is captured digitally and subjected to various analyses to extract biological information. Comparison of hybridization patterns enables the identification of mRNAs that differ in abundance in two or more target samples.[1,2]

Microarray technology was introduced in the 1990s, although the methods microarray-based were first conceived and developed in the 1980s.[3-6] Since then both commercial and academic groups have developed a number of different microarrays platforms and there are now numerous high-density platforms available which differ in terms of probe content, design, deposition technology, labeling and hybridization protocols. Regarding probe types, possible choices include spotted cDNA sequences or PCR products, and short or long oligonucleotides ranging from 25 to 70 base pair. However, two major platforms for high-density microarray manufacture are in common use (Fig. 1). Both methods share the feature of a solid support "chip" to which hundreds of thousands of gene fragments are attached.

*Susanna Mandruzzato—Oncology Section, Department Oncological and Surgical Sciences, University of Padova, Via Gattamelata 64, 35128 Padova, Italy.
Email: susanna.mandruzzato@unipd.it

Microarray Technology and Cancer Gene Profiling, edited by Simone Mocellin.
©2007 Landes Bioscience and Springer Science+Business Media.

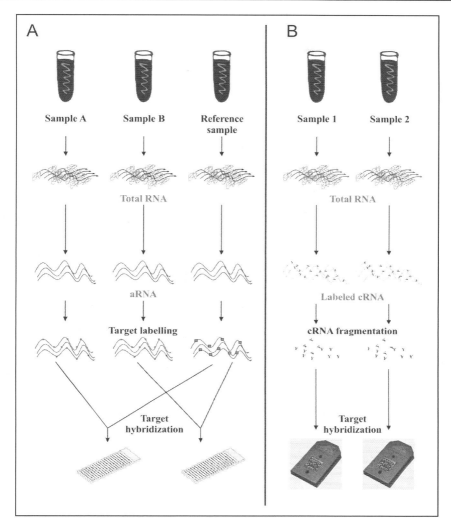

Figure 1. The two major microarray platforms. A) cDNA arrays. cDNA arrays are hybridized with two different targets derived from two samples to be compared. The two targets must be labeled with different fluorochromes and simultaneously hybridized with a glass microarray in a single reaction. B) Short oligonucleotide arrays. These arrays are one-channel arrays that give an absolute measurement of mRNA binding, that can be directly compared with the results of other oligonucleotide microarray experiments.

The first utilizes robotic deposition or "spotting" of DNA molecules that can be in the form of PCR-amplified complementary DNA (cDNA), presynthesized oligonucleotides, or genomic DNA like plasmids or bacterial artificial chromosomes (BAC). These spotted arrays are referred to as "cDNA microarrays".

The second technology was developed by Affymetrix™, using 25-mer oligonucleotides synthesized in situ by a photolithographic process similar to manufacture of computer chips in which up to 1.3 million different oligonucleotide probes are synthesized on each array. Each oligonucleotide is located in a specific area on the array called a probe cell and each probe cell contains hundreds of thousands to millions of copies of a given oligonucleotide.[3,7,8]

Beside the different immobilized probe used to detect specific mRNA transcripts, the main difference between the two types of arrays is the number of biological samples used within a single chip experiment. cDNA microarrays are two-channel arrays, with both a reference and experimental sample analyzed in the same chip. Samples are labeled with two fluorescent dyes, generally Cy3 (green) and Cy5 (red), and the chip scanner measures the amount of the two signals and eventually gives the ratio of the two intensities, therefore giving the result in terms of evaluation of a signal as compared to a "reference" sample (Fig. 1, panel A). Typical cDNA microarray experiments compare a normal cell or tissue samples to a treated or pathological sample.[2]

Oligonucleotide-based arrays are one-channel arrays that give an absolute measurement of mRNA binding, and this result can be directly compared with the results of other oligonucleotide microarray experiments (Fig. 1, panel B). The key point for this DNA array platform is the targeted design of probe sets. Using as little as 200 to 300 bases of gene, cDNA or EST sequence, independent 25-mer oligonucleotides are selected to serve as unique, sequence-specific detectors. The arrays are designed in silico, and as a result, it is not necessary to prepare, verify, quantitate and catalogue a large number of cDNAs, PCR products and clones, and there is no risk of a misidentified tube, clone, cDNA or spot. Although the binding of the probe to the target is constituted by an oligonucleotide long only 25 base pair, Affymetrix™ technology achieves a high grade of specificity by using for each probe set multiple probe pairs, consisting of perfect match (PM) oligonucleotides and corresponding mismatch (MM) oligonucleotides, used as control for nonspecific binding. For each probe designed to be perfectly complementary to a target sequence (PM), a partner probe is generated that is identical except for a single base mismatch in its center, the MM oligonucleotide (Fig. 2). This probe mismatch strategy, along with the use of multiple probes for each transcript, helps to identify and minimize the effects of nonspecific hybridization and background signal. Moreover, the use of multiple independent detectors for the same molecule greatly improves signal-to-noise ratios, improves the accuracy of RNA quantitation, reduces the effects of cross-hybridization, and drastically decreases the rate of false positives. In addition, short-chain oligonucleotides with single points of constraint are probably more accessible for hybridization to target than cDNA probes.

The latest generation of GeneChip expression arrays is represented by arrays with smaller feature size (11 microns), allowing the expression of all known transcripts of an organism to be analyzed on a single array.

Target Preparation and Hybridization

All the different platforms employing cDNA or oligonucleotide use unique target amplification and labeling protocols. It must be stressed that in every case the results of the assay are dependent upon the quality of the input RNA.

For eukaryotic samples, oligonucleotide-based arrays use double-stranded cDNA that is synthesized from total RNA or purified poly-A messenger RNA isolated from tissue or cells. Depending on the amount of starting material, two procedures can be used: the one-cycle or the two-cycle Eukaryotic Target Labeling. In the first case, total RNA (1 μg to 15 μg) or mRNA (0.2 μg to 2 μg) is first reverse transcribed in the first-strand cDNA synthesis reaction using the a reverse transcriptase, an oncoretroviral enzyme that uses RNA as a template for the synthesis of a single-stranded cDNA. This enzyme requires a short primer to initiate cDNA synthesis, and this is provided by an oligo(dT) promoter primer. Following RNase H-mediated second-strand cDNA synthesis, the double-stranded cDNA is purified and it is used as a template in the subsequent in vitro transcription (IVT) reaction. The GeneChip® 3'-Amplification reagents for IVT Labeling Kit is based on a T7 RNA polymerase-mediated reaction, optimized to start with as little as 1 μg of total RNA. This IVT reaction is carried out in the presence of a biotinylated nucleotide analog/ribonucleotide mix for complementary RNA (cRNA) amplification and biotin labeling. The biotinylated cRNA targets are then cleaned up, fragmented, and hybridized to GeneChip expression arrays.

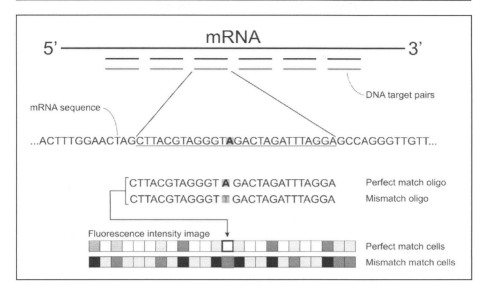

Figure 2. Oligonucleotide array scheme. Crucial for this approach is the use of target redundancy, which is not meant as the deposition of the same piece of DNA in multiple locations on an array, but rather the use of multiple oligonucleotides of different sequence designed to hybridize to different regions of the same RNA. For each gene monitored, several oligonucleotides are synthesized, using photolithography, directly on to the chip. Oligonucleotides are arranged as pairs: each pair includes a perfect match 25mer which is an exact complement to the gene sequence, and a control oligonucleotide, which differs from the perfect match oligo at the 13th base. The reported hybridization intensity is a composite of the different perfect match – mismatch differences per gene. This redundancy considerably increases the statistical power of the technology and data can be analyzed using standard statistical techniques, or by taking advantage of the changes in relative hybridization between perfect match and mismatch oligos to define genes as absent, present, increased or decreased according to a set of heuristic rules. The mismatch probes act as specificity controls that allow the direct subtraction of both background and cross-hybridization signals, and allow discrimination between "real" signals and those due to nonspecific or semi-specific hybridization, which are more likely to occur with single spot strategy DNA arrays (e.g., cDNA array platform). In the presence of even low concentrations of RNA, hybridization to the perfect match/mismatch pairs produces recognizable and quantitative fluorescent patterns. The strength of these patterns directly relates to the concentration of the RNA molecules in the complex sample (even without a competitive hybridization or two-color comparison).

For smaller amounts of starting total RNA, in the range of 10 ng to 100 ng, an additional cycle of cDNA synthesis and IVT amplification is required to obtain sufficient amounts of labeled cRNA target for analysis with arrays. After cDNA synthesis in the first cycle, an unlabeled ribonucleotide mix is used in the first cycle of IVT amplification. The unlabeled cRNA is then reverse transcribed in the first-strand cDNA synthesis step of the second cycle using random primers. Subsequently, the T7-Oligo(dT) Promoter Primer is used in the second-strand cDNA synthesis to generate double-stranded cDNA template containing T7 promoter sequences. The resulting double-stranded cDNA is then amplified and labeled using a biotinylated nucleotide analog/ribonucleotide mix in the second IVT reaction. The labeled cRNA is then cleaned up, fragmented with a buffer optimized to break down full-length cRNA to 35 to 200 base fragments by metal-induced hydrolysis. Eventually, the fragmented cRNA is hybridized to GeneChip expression arrays.

For prokaryotic samples, total RNA is isolated followed by reverse transcription with random hexamers to produce cDNA. The cDNA products are then fragmented by DNase I and labeled with terminal transferase and biotinylated GeneChip® DNA Labeling Reagent at the 3' termini. After determining that the fragmented cDNA is labeled with biotin, it is hybridized to the array.

To prepare the target for cDNA microarrays, sample RNA is converted to target by using the enzyme reverse transcriptase and usually by an oligo(dT), which anneals to the poly(A) tail found at the 3' end of the vast majority of mammalian mRNAs. The label incorporated into the cDNA can be either radioactive or fluorescent. Radioactive target is generated by incorporation of [33P]dCTP, and therefore this implies that comparison of different targets must be carried out using serial hybridizations to the same microarray or by parallel analyses using separate microarrays. An advantage of fluorescence detection is that competitive hybridization can be performed to the same microarray, and therefore can be used to compare targets derived from different samples. The relative hybridization of the targets labeled with different fluors to the same probe can be readily quantified. The fluorescent labels Cy3-dUTP and Cy5-dUTP are frequently paired, as they have high incorporation efficiencies with reverse transcriptase and good photostability and yield. Moreover, they are widely separated in their excitation and emission spectra, allowing highly discriminating optical filtration. RNA purity is a critical factor in hybridization performance, particularly when fluorescence is used, as cellular protein, lipid, and carbohydrate can mediate significant nonspecific binding of labeled cDNA to matrix surfaces.

A limitation of cDNA microarray technology is the large amount of RNA required to produce an adequate signal over noise. This is a critical issue with low-abundance transcripts. Fluorescence detection requires at least 10 μg of total RNA, whereas radioactive detection enables detection with as little as 0.1 μg of starting total RNA. To broaden the use of cDNA microarrays, some form of amplification process needs to be incorporated into the procedure. PCR is a highly efficient method for exponentially amplifying a population of single stranded cDNA. However, the nonlinear amplification results in a target in which sequence representation is skewed compared with the original mRNA pool. To overcome this problem, a linear amplification strategy of mRNA has been devised (see also the dedicated chapter in this book).[9,10]

cDNA arrays are hybridized with two different targets derived from two samples to be compared; when using fluorescent detection they must be labeled with different fluorochromes and simultaneously hybridized with a glass microarray in a single competitive reaction. Many RNA labeling protocols are currently employed for use with microarrays. The RNA can be labeled using reverse transcriptase to directly incorporate nucleotides covalently linked to fluorescent molecules. While this is the simplest method, the bulky fluorochromes do not always incorporate efficiently during the transcription, often resulting in biased incorporation of the Cy3- over the Cy5-labeled nucleotide. To overcome this problem, the cDNA can be indirectly labeled by enzymatic incorporation of amino allyl-modified and/or amino hexyl-modified nucleotides into the cDNA followed by chemical coupling of the Cy3 and Cy5 fluors to the amino allyl/hexyl groups. This labeling is more efficient and less biased than direct incorporation labeling as the amino allyl/hexyl groups are smaller and less bulky than the fluorescent nucleotide molecules.

Eventually the competitive hybridization between these two RNA molecules is analyzed by comparing the ratio of the intensity of the two fluorochromes such as Cy3 and Cy5 (Fig. 3). Because a ratio is used, experimental results can be compared across multiple arrays despite slight variations in the DNA concentration on the array from different print sets.

Image Acquisition and Quantification

After the hybridization step is complete, and the probe array is washed and stained, the microarray is placed in a scanner, in which the fluorescent tags are excited by a laser and a digital image of the array is created.

In the oligonucleotide-based array system, an image file is generated. In the first step of the analysis, a grid is automatically placed over the file demarcating each probe cell. The software defines the probe cells and computes an intensity for each cell. A statistical algorithm then

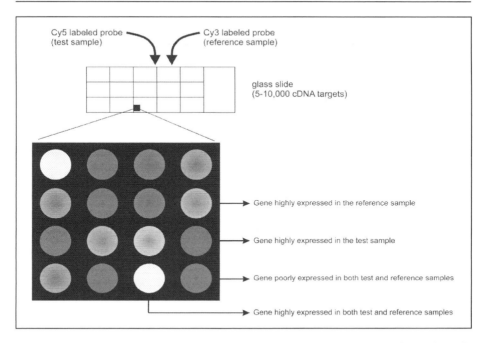

Figure 3. Scheme of glass-based cDNA array. DNA targets are represented by cDNA clones robotically spotted onto a solid surface. Each spot on the array represents a portion of a gene. DNA probes derive from reverse transcribed RNA extracted from biological samples. Typically, two probes are hybridized on a single array: they are the control probe (usually labeled with Cy3 fluorophore) and the experimental probe (usually labeled with Cy5 fluorophore). The transcriptional levels of a given gene in an experimental situation is therefore expressed as a relative ratio with respect with the control sample. The resulting image is produced by superimposing the Cy3 fluorescence image (pseudocolored green) and the Cy5 fluorescence image (pseudocolored red). Thus, red, green and yellow colors represent respectively increased, decreased and equal gene copy number in the experimental sample with respect to the control sample. Low fluorescence intensity is due to low gene expression in both samples. A color version of this figure is available online at www.Eurekah.com.

generates a detection *p*-value to determine the detection call which indicates whether a transcript is reliably detected (Present) or not detected (Absent). Additionally, a signal value is calculated which assigns a relative measure of abundance to the transcript.

As regards cDNA microarrays, once targets have been hybridized to probes and the microarray has been washed to remove as much unbound and nonspecifically bound target as possible, the array must be scanned to determine how much target is bound to each probe spot. Data are captured from microarrays hybridized with ^{33}P-labeled target by means of a phosphorimager system. Microarrays hybridized with fluorescent targets are stimulated with a laser and the emitted light is then captured by a confocal scanner (Fig. 3). A number of companies produce machines for scanning fluorescently labeled microarrays. Image quantification is then performed using the associated software, and the amount of mRNA bound to the spots on the microarray is precisely measured, generating a profile of gene expression in the sample. This program can either calculate the red-to-green fluorescence ratio or to subtract out background data for each microarray spot by analyzing the digital image of the array. A table containing the ratios of the intensity of red-to-green fluorescence for every spot on the array is then created.

References

1. Southern E, Mir K, Shchepinov M. Molecular interactions on microarrays. Nat Genet 1999; 21(1 Suppl):5-9.
2. Duggan DJ et al. Expression profiling using cDNA microarrays. Nat Genet 1999; 21(1 Suppl):10-4.
3. Fodor SP et al. Light-directed, spatially addressable parallel chemical synthesis. Science 1991; 251(4995):767-73.
4. Maskos U, Southern EM. Parallel analysis of oligodeoxyribonucleotide (oligonucleotide) interactions. I. Analysis of factors influencing oligonucleotide duplex formation. Nucleic Acids Res 1992; 20(7):1675-8.
5. Schena M et al. Quantitative monitoring of gene expression patterns with a complementary DNA microarray. Science 1995; 270(5235):467-70.
6. Ekins R, Chu F, Micallef J. High specific activity chemiluminescent and fluorescent markers: Their potential application to high sensitivity and 'multi-analyte' immunoassays. J Biolumin Chemilumin 1989; 4(1):59-78.
7. Fodor SP et al. Multiplexed biochemical assays with biological chips. Nature 1993; 364(6437):555-6.
8. Pease AC et al. Light-generated oligonucleotide arrays for rapid DNA sequence analysis. Proc Natl Acad Sci USA 1994; 91(11):5022-6.
9. Wang E et al. High-fidelity mRNA amplification for gene profiling. Nat Biotechnol 2000; 18(4):457-9.
10. Feldman AL et al. Advantages of mRNA amplification for microarray analysis. Biotechniques 2002; 33(4):906-12, 914.

CHAPTER 3

Principles of Gene Microarray Data Analysis

Simone Mocellin* and Carlo Riccardo Rossi

Abstract

The development of several gene expression profiling methods, such as comparative genomic hybridization (CGH), differential display, serial analysis of gene expression (SAGE), and gene microarray, together with the sequencing of the human genome, has provided an opportunity to monitor and investigate the complex cascade of molecular events leading to tumor development and progression. The availability of such large amounts of information has shifted the attention of scientists towards a nonreductionist approach to biological phenomena. High throughput technologies can be used to follow changing patterns of gene expression over time. Among them, gene microarray has become prominent because it is easier to use, does not require large-scale DNA sequencing, and allows for the parallel quantification of thousands of genes from multiple samples. Gene microarray technology is rapidly spreading worldwide and has the potential to drastically change the therapeutic approach to patients affected with tumor. Therefore, it is of paramount importance for both researchers and clinicians to know the principles underlying the analysis of the huge amount of data generated with microarray technology.

Introduction

The advent of the genome project has vastly increased our knowledge of the genomic sequences of humans and other organisms, as well as the genes that they encode. Various techniques have been developed to exploit this growing body of data, including serial analysis of gene expression (SAGE)[1] and gene microarray,[2] which provide rapid, parallel surveys of gene-expression patterns for hundreds or thousands of genes in a single assay. These transcriptional profiling techniques promise a wealth of data that can be used to develop a more complete understanding of gene function, regulation and interactions. The most powerful applications of transcriptional profiling involve the study of patterns of gene expression across many experiments that survey a wide array of cellular responses, phenotypes and conditions. The simplest way to identify genes of potential interest through several related experiments is to search for those that are consistently either up- or downregulated. To that end, a simple statistical analysis of gene-expression levels will suffice. However, identifying patterns of gene expression and grouping genes into expression classes might provide much greater insight into their biological function and relevance. Several techniques have been used for the analysis of gene-expression data. The implementation of a successful program of expression analysis requires the development of various laboratory protocols, as well as the development of database and software tools for efficient data collection and analysis. Although detailed laboratory

*Corresponding Author: Simone Mocellin—Clinica Chirurgica II, Dipartimento di Scienze Oncologiche e Chirurgiche, University of Padova, Via Giustiniani 2, Padova, Italy. Email: mocellins@hotmail.com

Microarray Technology and Cancer Gene Profiling, edited by Simone Mocellin.
©2007 Landes Bioscience and Springer Science+Business Media.

protocols have been published, the computational tools necessary to analyze the data are rapidly evolving and no clear consensus exists as to the best method for revealing patterns of gene expression. Indeed, it is becoming increasingly clear that there might never be a "best" approach and that the application of various techniques will allow different aspects of the data to be explored. Furthermore, without a more complete understanding of the underlying biology, particularly of gene regulation, there might never be a single technique that will allow us to find all the relationships in the data. Consequently, choosing the appropriate algorithms for analysis is a crucial element of the experimental design.

The purpose of this chapter is to provide readers with a general overview of some existing computational approaches. This chapter is not comprehensive, as new, more sophisticated techniques are rapidly being developed, but instead represents a tutorial on some of the more basic tools. Although the focus here is on spotted cDNA microarrays,[3] the techniques described are generally applicable to expression data generated using oligonucleotide arrays[4] or SAGE, provided that data are presented in an appropriate format.

Study Design and Data Analysis

The correlation observed between gene expression levels from duplicate spots on a single array usually exceeds 95%. This is often interpreted as a demonstration of reproducibility. However, if the same sample is split and hybridized to two different arrays, the correlation across hybridizations is likely to fall to the 60 to 80% range. Correlations between samples obtained from individual inbred mice may be as low as 30%. If the experiments are carried out in different laboratories, the correlations may be even lower. These decreasing correlations reflect the cumulative contributions of multiple sources of variation.[5] The main sources of variability are biological and technical variation. As for the former, it is generally appropriate to take steps to vary the conditions of the experiment—for example, by assaying multiple animals —to ensure that the effects that do achieve statistical significance are real and will be reproducible in different settings.

Identifying the independent units in an experiment is a prerequisite for a proper statistical analysis, as any hidden correlations in the data can lead to bias and inflated levels of statistical significance. In general, two measurements may be regarded as independent only if the experimental materials on which the measurements were obtained could have received different treatments, and if the materials were handled separately at all stages of the experiment where variation might have been introduced. For instance, consider a cell line that is divided into eight equal samples. Four are assigned to one treatment, and the remaining four receive a second treatment. The eight aliquots are handled separately throughout the entire experimental procedure, and each is measured in triplicate. This results in 24 total observations, but there are eight experimental units. Now consider a cell line that is divided into two aliquots, each one receiving a different treatment. The material is further subdivided into four aliquots per treatment group, each of which is processed and then measured in triplicate. Again we have 24 observations, but now there are only two independent experimental units.

A simple way to assess the adequacy of a design is to determine the degrees of freedom (df). This is done by counting the number of independent units and subtracting from it the number of distinct treatments (count all combinations that occur if there are multiple treatment factors). If there are no degrees of freedom left, there may be no information available to estimate the biological variance, and the statistical tests will rely on technical variance alone. Five df or more are generally recommended for a statistical analysis to be considered sound (Fig. 1).

In order to increase DNA array result reproducibility, the issue of technical variability should also be addressed while designing experiments. Although this can be achieved by repeating the experiment, high throughput DNA array experts suggest that the use of spot replicates within the same array is the best way to deal with this issue.[6,7] In particular, biostatistical analysis has shown that a minimum of three replicates should be used to reduce the number of false positive and false negative results generated by studies performed without replication.[8]

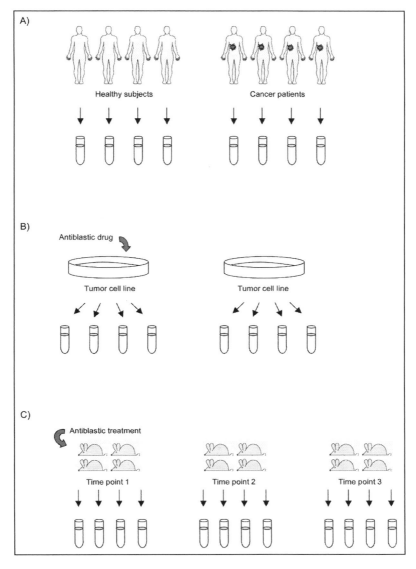

Figure 1. Study design for DNA array-based experiments. A) Pairwise comparison. In the search for carcino-genesis related genes, the gene profile of tumor biopsies from 4 patients is compared to that of normal tissue biopsies from 4 healthy subjects, providing 6 (8 independent experimental units minus 2 experimental conditions) residual degrees of freedom (df). B) In this experiment, the gene profile of two samples (one treated with an antiblastic drug) of the same tumor cell line are compared in order to dissect the mechanism of action of the antiblastic drug. Four aliquots are obtained from each cell line and directly compared on pairs of DNA arrays. The experiment lacks biological replication because the aliquots are not independent (2 independent experimental units, 2 treatments, df = 0). The design could be improved by using 8 independent cell lines, 4 of them treated with the antiblastic agent (in this case df would be 6). C) In a time course study on the effects of an antiblastic treatment on the gene profile of the tumor microenvironment, 3 time points are considered, 4 mice being sampled from each of them (12 independent experimental units, 3 experimental conditions, df = 9).

Comparison of Independent and Paired Samples

The comparison of two independent samples (e.g., diseased versus normal tissue) is the simplest experimental situation. Although a number of statistical tests are available to assess the significance of the observed differences, most of the groups active in this field use filtering rules based on arbitrarily assigned fold difference criteria. This strategy lies on the unverified assumption that a less than X-fold difference in gene expression is not associated with a significant biological effect. Despite the good results yielded with this method,[3,9,10] it is possible that the application of a simple fold-based rule leads to false positive results.[11] Classical statistical techniques can be adopted to test the significance of the observed differences.[12,13] For example, if two independent samples are compared, a standard t-test is appropriate. The genes in the array can be ranked according to increasing P values and an appropriate threshold can be chosen depending on the percentage of false positives that we are prepared to tolerate. If the two samples to be compared are somehow related with each other (i.e., they both come from the same individual) then a paired t-test would be needed to assess the significance of the differences. More complex experimental situations may involve the comparison of multiple samples. Appropriate statistical tests are available, but in analogy with the two-sample comparison case, threshold rules are often employed.[11]

Classification of Gene Expression Data

Gene microarrays deliver several thousands of measurements per experiment. The analysis, interpretation, and meaningful display and storage of such a large volume of data is particularly challenging. Although genes that display extreme expression changes between samples may require specific analysis, the true strength of high-throughput experiments in revealing the complexity of tumor/host relation derives from the mathematical identification of expression patterns (called "signatures") within profiling data. In the context of gene expression studies, this involves finding similar gene expression patterns by comparing profiles. Dedicated software developed for this task includes the "unsupervised" and "supervised" varieties.[14] Unsupervised methods (e.g., cluster analysis,[15] self organizing map (SOM),[16] principal component analysis (PCA)[17] define classes without any a priori intervention on data, which are organized by clustering genes and/or samples simply according to similarities in their expression profiles. The resulting sample classification often correlates with a general characteristic of the sample as defined by large sets of genes and not necessarily with the particular feature of interest, generally identified by a smaller set of genes. By defining relevant classes before analysis, supervised techniques (e.g., support vector machines,[18] weighted votes,[19] and neural networks[20]) bypass this issue. These algorithms incorporate external information related to samples studied to identify the optimal set of genes that best discriminate between experimental samples. Unsupervised clustering techniques for analyzing microarrays are useful for initial data exploration, and have been validated under certain circumstances by their successful "rediscovery" of known classes of genes. In particular, unsupervised techniques can be effectively adopted in oncology when the aim of the study is to identify new prognostic subgroups.[21] However, these methods have certain shortfalls. Since prior biological knowledge is not incorporated, all measurements within the expression profile contribute equally to the analysis. Thus measurements that have little or nothing to do with distinguishing the groups of interest can confound the placement of an example into the correct category. The advantage of supervised classification for gene profile analysis is its ability to incorporate biological knowledge. For example, a supervised approach might be used to predict whether a gene's product is involved in protein synthesis by comparing its expression profile to the profiles of both genes known to be involved and genes known not to be involved in protein synthesis. Yet, recent reports have demonstrated the ability of supervised classification to subtype leukemia (myeloid versus lymphoid)[19] and assign functions to genes[22] based on gene microarray data.

Data Collection and Normalization

Once a collection of microarray slides is printed, each slide represents a potential experiment. The arrayed genes are probes that can be used to query pooled, differentially labeled targets derived from RNA samples from different cellular phenotypes to determine the relative expression levels of each gene. The two RNA samples from the tissues of interest are typically used to generate first-strand cDNA targets labeled with the fluorescent dyes Cy3 and Cy5. These are then purified, pooled and hybridized to the arrays. After hybridization, slides are scanned and independent images for the control and query channels are generated. These images must then be analyzed to identify the arrayed spots and to measure the relative fluorescence intensities for each element.

After image processing, it is necessary to normalize the relative fluorescence intensities in each of the two scanned channels. Normalization adjusts for differences in labeling and detection efficiencies for the fluorescent labels and for differences in the quantity of initial RNA from the two samples examined in the assay. These problems can cause a shift in the average ratio of Cy5 to Cy3 and the intensities must be rescaled before an experiment can be properly analyzed. There are three widely used techniques that can be used to normalize gene-expression data from single array hybridization: (1) total intensity normalization, (2) normalization using regression techniques, and (3) normalization using ratio statistics. All of these assume that all (or most) of the genes in the array, some subset of genes, or a set of exogenous controls that have been "spiked" into the RNA before labeling, should have an average expression ratio equal to one. The normalization factor is then used to adjust the data to compensate for experimental variability and to "balance" the fluorescence signals from the two samples being compared.

Total intensity normalization data relies on the assumption that the quantity of initial mRNA is the same for both labeled samples. Furthermore, one assumes that some genes are upregulated in the query sample relative to the control and that others are downregulated. For the hundreds or thousands of genes in the array, these changes should balance out so that the total quantity of RNA hybridizing to the array from each sample is the same. Consequently, the total integrated intensity computed for all the elements in the array should be the same in both the Cy3 and Cy5 channels. Under this assumption, a normalization factor can be calculated and used to rescale the intensity for each gene in the array.

The second normalization method hinges upon regression techniques. For mRNA derived from closely related samples, a significant fraction of the assayed genes are expected to be expressed at similar levels. In a scatter plot of Cy5 versus Cy3 intensities (or their logarithms), these genes would cluster along a straight line, the slope of which would be one if the labeling and detection efficiencies were the same for both samples. Normalization of these data is equivalent to calculating the best-fit slope using regression techniques and adjusting the intensities so that the calculated slope is one. In many experiments, the intensities are nonlinear, and local regression techniques are more suitable, such as LOWESS (LOcally WEighted Scatterplot Smoothing) regression.

A third normalization option is a method based on the ratio statistics. They assume that although individual genes might be up- or downregulated, in closely related cells, the total quantity of RNA produced is approximately the same for essential genes, such as "housekeeping genes". Using this assumption, they develop an approximate probability density for the ratio $Tk = Rk/Gk$ (where Rk and Gk are, respectively, the measured red and green intensities for the kth array element). They then describe how this can be used in an iterative process that normalizes the mean expression ratio to one and calculates confidence limits that can be used to identify differentially expressed genes.

After normalization, the data for each gene are typically reported as an "expression ratio" or as the logarithm of the expression ratio. The expression ratio is simply the normalized value of the expression level for a particular gene in the query sample divided by its normalized value for the control. The advantage of using the logarithm of the expression ratio is simple to understand. Genes that are upregulated by a factor of 2 have an expression ratio of 2, whereas those downregulated by the same factor have an expression ratio of one-half (0.5), which implies that downregulated genes are "squashed" between 1 and 0. By contrast, a gene upregulated by a factor of 2 has a log2(ratio) of 1, whereas a gene downregulated by a factor of 2 has a log2(ratio) of -1, and a gene expressed at a constant level (with a ratio of 1) has a log2(ratio) of 0. At this point in the analysis of a single experiment, we typically look for genes that are differentially expressed. Most published studies have used a post-normalization cut-off of twofold increase or decrease in measured level to define differential expression, although there is no firm theoretical basis for selecting this level as significant.

It should be noted that there are disadvantages to using only expression ratios for data analysis. Although ratios can help to reveal some patterns in the data, they remove all information about the absolute gene-expression levels. Various parameters depend on the measured intensity, including the confidence limits that are placed on any microarray measurement. Although most of the techniques developed for analysis of microarray data use ratios, many of them can be adapted for use with measured intensities.

Comparing Expression Data

The true power of microarray analysis does not come from the analysis of single experiments, but rather, from the analysis of many hybridizations to identify common patterns of gene expression. Based on our understanding of cellular processes, genes that are contained in a particular pathway, or that respond to a common environmental challenge, should be coregulated and consequently, should show similar patterns of expression. Our goal then is to identify genes that show similar patterns of expression and there exists a large group of statistical methods, generally referred to as "cluster analysis" (the term "cluster analysis" actually encompasses several different classification algorithms that can be used to develop taxonomies, typically as part of exploratory data analysis) that can be used to achieve this.

For expression data, we can begin to address the problem of "similarity" mathematically by defining an "expression vector" for each gene that represents its location in "expression space". In this view of gene expression, each experiment represents a separate, distinct axis in space and the log2(ratio) measured for that gene in that experiment represents its geometric coordinate. For example, if we have three experiments, the log2(ratio) for a given gene in experiment 1 is its *x* coordinate, the log2(ratio) in experiment 2 is its *y* coordinate, and the log2(ratio) in experiment 3 is its *z* coordinate. So, we can represent all the information we have about that gene by a point in *x*–*y*–*z*-expression space. A second gene, with nearly the same log2(ratio) values for each experiment will be represented by a (spatially) nearby point in expression space; a gene with a very different pattern of expression will be far from our original gene. The generalization to more experiments is straightforward (although harder to draw): the dimensionality of expression space grows to be equal to the number of experiments. In this way, expression data can be represented in *n*-dimensional expression space, where *n* is the number of experiments, and where each gene-expression vector is represented as a single point in that space. Having been provided with a means of measuring distance between genes, clustering algorithms sort the data and group genes together on the basis of their separation in expression space. It should also be noted that if we are interested in clustering experiments, we could represent each experiment as an "experiment vector" consisting of the expression values for each gene; these define an "experiment space", the dimensionality of which is equal to the number of genes assayed in each experiment. Again, by defining distances appropriately, we could apply any of the clustering algorithms defined here to analyze and group experiments. To interpret the results from any analysis of multiple experiments, it is helpful to have an intuitive visual representation. A commonly used approach relies on the creation of an expression matrix in which each column of the matrix represents a single experiment and each row represents the expression vector for a particular gene. Coloring each of the matrix elements on the basis of its expression value creates a visual representation of gene-expression patterns across the collection of experiments. There are countless ways in which the expression matrix can be colored and presented. The most commonly used method colors genes on the basis of their log2(ratio) in each experiment, with log2(ratio) values close to zero colored black, those with log2(ratio) values greater than zero colored red, and those with negative values colored green. For each element in the matrix, the relative intensity represents the relative expression, with brighter elements being more highly differentially expressed. For any particular group of experiments, the expression matrix generally appears without any apparent pattern or order. Programs designed to cluster data generally reorder the rows, or columns, or both, such that patterns of expression become visually apparent when presented in this fashion.

Before clustering the data, there are two further questions that need to be considered: first, should the data be adjusted in some way to enhance certain relationships? And second, what distance measure should be used to group together related genes? In many microarray experiments, the data analysis can be dominated by the variables that have the largest values, obscuring other, important differences. One way to circumvent this problem is to adjust or rescale the data and there are several methods in common use with microarray data. For example, each vector can be rescaled so that the average expression of each gene is zero, a process referred to as "mean centering". In this process, the basal expression level of a gene is subtracted from each experimental measurement. This has the effect of enhancing the variation of the expression pattern of each gene across experiments, without regard to whether the gene is primarily up- or downregulated. This is particularly useful for the analysis of time-course experiments, in which one might like to find genes that show similar variation around their basal expression level. The data can also be adjusted so that the minimum and maximum are ± 1, or so that the "length" of each expression vector is one. The manner in which we measure distance between gene-expression vectors also has a profound effect on the clusters that are produced.

Clustering Algorithms

Various clustering techniques have been applied to the identification of patterns in gene-expression data. Most cluster analysis techniques are hierarchical; the resultant classification has an increasing number of nested classes and the result resembles a phylogenetic classification. Nonhierarchical clustering techniques also exist, such as k-means clustering, which simply partition objects into different clusters without trying to specify the relationship between individual elements. Clustering techniques can further be classified as divisive or agglomerative. A divisive method begins with all elements in one cluster that is gradually broken down into smaller and smaller clusters. Agglomerative techniques start with (usually) single-member clusters and gradually fuse them together. Finally, clustering can be either supervised or unsupervised. Supervised methods use existing biological information about specific genes that are functionally related to "guide" the clustering algorithm. However, most methods are unsupervised and these are dealt with first.

Unsupervised Methods

Hierarchical Clustering

Hierarchical clustering has the advantage that it is simple and the result can be easily visualized. It has become one of the most widely used techniques for the analysis of gene-expression data. Hierarchical clustering is an agglomerative approach in which single expression profiles are joined to form groups, which are further joined until the process has been carried to completion, forming a single hierarchical tree (Fig. 2). The process of hierarchical clustering proceeds in a simple manner. First, the pairwise distance matrix is calculated for all of the genes to be clustered. Second, the distance matrix is searched for the two most similar genes (see above) or clusters; initially each cluster consists of a single gene. This is the first true stage in the "clustering"

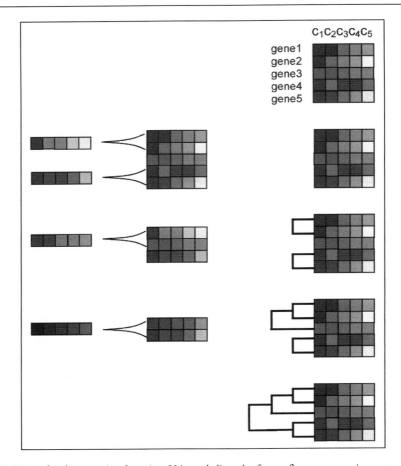

Figure 2. Hierarchical aggregative clustering. Using a dedicated software, fluorescence ratios are translated into color codes. Consequently, genes with unchanged expression levels are colored as black, while those with increasingly positive or negative expression are colored with increasingly intense red or green, respectively. Accordingly, the darker the color, the closer to unchanged expression. The figure shows an example with the color coded expression values of five genes in five different experimental conditions (c1, c2, c3, c4, c5). In the aggregative method, the closest pair of profiles is chosen based on a given metric. Then, an average of both profiles is constructed. This defines a relationship of closeness between both profiles that remain tied by the corresponding branch of the tree. Thus, the linked profiles are substituted by the average profile and the process continues until all the profiles are linked. The linkage relationship defines the hierarchy of the tree.

process. If several pairs have the same separation distance, a predetermined rule is used to decide between alternatives. Third, the two selected clusters are merged to produce a new cluster that now contains at least two objects. Fourth, the distances are calculated between this new cluster and all other clusters. There is no need to calculate all distances as only those involving the new cluster have changed. Last, steps 2–4 are repeated until all objects are in one cluster. There are several variations on hierarchical clustering that differ in the rules governing how distances are measured between clusters as they are constructed. They include, but are not limited to:

　　1. Single-linkage clustering. The distance between two clusters, i and j, is calculated as the minimum distance between a member of cluster i and a member of cluster j. Consequently,

this technique is also referred to as the minimum, or nearest-neighbor, method. This method tends to produce clusters that are "loose" because clusters can be joined if any two members are close together. In particular, this method often results in "chaining", or the sequential addition of single samples to an existing cluster. This produces trees with many long, single-addition branches representing clusters that have grown by accretion.

2. Complete-linkage clustering. This type of clustering is also known as the maximum or furthest-neighbor method. The distance between two clusters is calculated as the greatest distance between members of the relevant clusters. Not surprisingly, this method tends to produce very compact clusters of elements and the clusters are often very similar in size.

3. Average-linkage clustering. The distance between clusters is calculated using average values. There are, in fact, various methods for calculating averages. The most common is the unweighted pair-group method average (UPGMA). The average distance is calculated from the distance between each point in a cluster and all other points in another cluster. The two clusters with the lowest average distance are joined together to form a new cluster. Related methods substitute the CENTROID (the centroid of a cluster is the weighted average point in the multidimensional space; in a sense, it is the center of gravity for the respective cluster) or the median for the average.

4. Weighted pair-group average. This method is identical to UPGMA, except for the fact that in the computations the size of the respective clusters (i.e., the number of objects contained in them) is used as a weight. This method (rather than UPGMA) should be used when the cluster sizes are suspected to be greatly uneven.

5. Within-groups clustering. This is similar to UPGMA except that clusters are merged and a cluster average is used for further calculations rather than the individual cluster elements. This tends to produce tighter clusters than UPGMA.

6. Ward's method. Cluster membership is determined by calculating the total sum of squared deviations from the mean of a cluster and joining clusters in such a manner that it produces the smallest possible increase in the sum of squared errors.

Each of these will produce slightly different results, as will any of the algorithms if the distance metric is changed. Typically for gene-expression data, average linkage clustering gives acceptable results. One potential problem with many hierarchical clustering methods is that, as clusters grow in size, the expression vector that represents the cluster might no longer represent any of the genes in the cluster. Consequently, as clustering progresses, the actual expression patterns of the genes themselves become less relevant. Furthermore, if a bad assignment is made early in the process, it cannot be corrected. An alternative, which can avoid these artifacts, is to use a divisive clustering approach, such as *k*-means or self-organizing maps, to partition data (either genes or experiments) into groups that have similar expression patterns.

K-Means Clustering

If there is advanced knowledge about the number of clusters that should be represented in the data, k-means clustering is a good alternative to hierarchical methods. In k-means clustering, objects are partitioned into a fixed number (k) of clusters, so that the clusters are internally similar but externally dissimilar. No dendrogram (i.e., a branching "tree" diagram representing a hierarchy of categories on the basis of degree of similarity or number of shared characteristics: the results of hierarchical clustering are presented as dendrograms, in which the distance along the tree from one element to the next represents their relative degree of similarity) is produced (but one could use hierarchical techniques on each of the data partitions after they are constructed). The process involved in k-means clustering is conceptually simple, but can be computationally intensive. First, all initial objects are randomly assigned to one of k clusters (where k is specified by the user). Second, an average expression vector is then calculated for each cluster and this is used to compute the distances between clusters. Third, using an iterative method, objects are moved between clusters and intra- and inter-cluster distances are measured with each move. Objects are allowed to remain in the new cluster only if they are closer to it than to their previous cluster. Fourth, after each move, the expression vectors for each cluster are recalculated. Last, the shuffling proceeds until moving any more objects would make the clusters more variable, increasing intra-cluster distances and decreasing inter-cluster dissimilarity. Some implementations of k-means clustering allow not only the number of clusters, but also seed cases (or genes) for each cluster, to be specified. This has the potential to allow, for example, use of previous knowledge of the system to help define the cluster output. For example, an attempt to classify patients with two histologically identical but clinically distinct (opposite prognosis or response to treatment) cancers using microarray expression patterns can be imagined. By using k-means clustering on experiments with k = 2, the data will be partitioned into two groups. The challenge then faced is to determine whether there are really only two distinct groups represented in the data or not. In this case, k-means clustering is particularly useful with other techniques, such as principal component analysis (PCA). PCA allows visual estimation of the number of clusters represented in the data. This can be used to specify k and to group genes (or experiments) into related clusters.

Principal Component Analysis

An analysis of microarray data is a search for genes that have similar, correlated patterns of expression. This indicates that some of the data might contain redundant information. For example, if a group of experiments were more closely related than we had expected, we could ignore some of the redundant experiments, or use some average of the information without loss of information. PCA is a mathematical technique that exploits these factors to pick out patterns in the data, while reducing the effective dimensionality of gene-expression space without significant loss of information. PCA is one of a family of related techniques that include factor analysis, which provides a "projection" of complex data sets onto a reduced, easily visualized space. Although the mathematics is complex, the basic principles are straightforward. Imagine taking a three-dimensional cloud of data points and rotating it so that you can view it from different perspectives. You might imagine that certain views would allow you to better separate the data into groups than other views. PCA finds those views that give you the best separation of the data. This technique can be applied to both genes and experiments as a means of classification. In most implementations of PCA, it is difficult to define accurately the precise boundaries of distinct clusters in the data, or to define genes (or experiments) belonging to each cluster. However, PCA is a powerful technique for the analysis of gene-expression data when used with another classification technique, such as k-means clustering or self-organizing maps (SOM), which require the user to specify the number of clusters.

Self-Organizing Maps

A SOM is a neural network-based divisive clustering approach. A SOM assigns genes to a series of partitions on the basis of the similarity of their expression vectors to reference vectors that are defined for each partition. It is the process of defining these reference vectors that distinguishes SOM from k-means clustering. Before initiating the analysis, the user defines a geometric configuration for the partitions, typically a two-dimensional rectangular or hexagonal grid. Random vectors are generated for each partition, but before genes can be assigned to partitions, the vectors are first "trained" using an iterative process that continues until convergence so that the data are most effectively separated. First, random vectors are constructed and assigned to each partition. Second, a gene is picked at random and, using a selected distance metric, the reference vector that is closest to the gene is identified. Third, the reference vector is then adjusted so that it is more similar to the vector of the assigned gene. The reference vectors that are nearby on the two-dimensional grid are also adjusted so that they are more similar to the vector of the assigned gene. Fourth, steps 2 and 3 are iterated several thousand times, decreasing the amount by which the reference vectors are adjusted and increasing the stringency used to define closeness in each step. As the process continues, the reference vectors converge to fixed values. Last, the genes are mapped to the relevant partitions depending on the reference vector to which they are most similar. In choosing the geometric configuration for the clusters, the user is, effectively, specifying the number of partitions into which the data is to be divided. As with k-means clustering, the user has to rely on some other source of information, such as PCA, to determine the number of clusters that best represents the available data.

Supervised Methods

The techniques discussed so far are unsupervised methods for identifying patterns of gene expression. Supervised methods represent a powerful alternative that can be applied if one has some previous information about which genes are expected to cluster together. One widely used example is the support vector machine (SVM).[22] SVM uses a training set in which genes known to be related by, for example function, provided as positive examples and genes known not to be members of that class are negative examples. These are combined into a set of training examples that is used by the SVM to learn to distinguish between members and nonmembers of the class on the basis of expression data. Having learned the expression features of the class, the SVM can then be used to recognize and classify the genes in the data set on the basis of their expression. In this way, SVM uses biological information to determine expression features that are characteristic of a group and to assign genes to that group. The SVM can also identify genes in the training set that are outliers or that have been previously assigned to the incorrect class.

As discussed previously, gene-expression data can be thought of as an m-dimensional space, in which expression vectors are represented as points in that space. An SVM is a binary classifier that attempts to separate genes into two classes (in the positive training set, or outside it) by defining an optimal HYPERPLANE separating class members from nonmembers. However, for most real examples, there is no simple solution to this problem in expression space. SVM solves the problem by mapping the gene-expression vectors from expression space into a higher-dimensional "feature space", in which distance is measured using a mathematical function known as a "kernel function" (a generalization of the distance metric: it measures the distance between two expression vectors as the data are projected into higher-dimensional space), and the data can then be separated into two classes. For some data sets, SVM might not achieve clean separation, either because of errors in classification in the training set, or noise in the data, or an improperly chosen kernel function. For this reason, most implementations also allow users to specify a "soft margin" that allows some training examples to fall on the wrong side of the separating hyperplane (an N-dimensional analogy of a line or plane that divides an "$N + 1$" dimensional space into two). Completely specifying a SVM therefore requires specifying both the kernel function and the magnitude of the penalty (usually called "cost") to be applied for violating the soft margin. As with the other techniques described here, this is one of the challenges of using SVM. It is often difficult to choose the best kernel function, parameters and penalties. Different parameters often yield completely different classifications. It is therefore often necessary to successively increase kernel complexity until an appropriate classification is achieved.

SVM are one of a group of supervised algorithms that have been applied to the classification of gene expression patterns. Although they might be of use in the identification of genes that share related expression patterns, an application of potentially greater impact is the use of supervised methods for the classification of samples. If we measure gene-expression patterns using RNA collected from various patients for which there is, for example, tumor-stage classification or survival data, we can use the microarray data to "train" an algorithm that can then be applied to the classification of other previously unclassified samples. This approach could lead to the development of "molecular expression fingerprinting" for tumor classification, in terms of both diagnosis and prognosis.[23]

References

1. Velculescu VE, Zhang L, Vogelstein B et al. Serial analysis of gene expression. Science 1995; 270(5235):484-7.
2. Brown PO, Botstein D. Exploring the new world of the genome with DNA microarrays. Nat Genet 1999; 21(1 Suppl):33-7.
3. Schena M, Shalon D, Davis RW et al. Quantitative monitoring of gene expression patterns with a complementary DNA microarray. Science 1995; 270(5235):467-70.
4. Lockhart DJ, Dong H, Byrne MC et al. Expression monitoring by hybridization to high-density oligonucleotide arrays. Nat Biotechnol 1996; 14(13):1675-80.
5. Churchill GA. Fundamentals of experimental design for cDNA microarrays. Nat Genet 2002; 32(Suppl):490-5.
6. Dopazo J, Zanders E, Dragoni I et al. Methods and approaches in the analysis of gene expression data. J Immunol Methods 2001; 250(1-2):93-112.
7. Hess KR, Zhang W, Baggerly KA et al. Microarrays: Handling the deluge of data and extracting reliable information. Trends Biotechnol 2001; 19(11):463-8.
8. Lee ML, Kuo FC, Whitmore GA et al. Importance of replication in microarray gene expression studies: Statistical methods and evidence from repetitive cDNA hybridizations. Proc Natl Acad Sci USA 2000; 97(18):9834-9.
9. Heller RA, Schena M, Chai A et al. Discovery and analysis of inflammatory disease-related genes using cDNA microarrays. Proc Natl Acad Sci USA 1997; 94(6):2150-5.
10. Teague TK, Hildeman D, Kedl RM et al. Activation changes the spectrum but not the diversity of genes expressed by T cells. Proc Natl Acad Sci USA 1999; 96(22):12691-6.
11. Claverie JM. Computational methods for the identification of differential and coordinated gene expression. Hum Mol Genet 1999; 8(10):1821-32.
12. Glynne R, Akkaraju S, Healy JI et al. How self-tolerance and the immunosuppressive drug FK506 prevent B-cell mitogenesis. Nature 2000; 403(6770):672-6.
13. Rogge L, Bianchi E, Biffi M et al. Transcript imaging of the development of human T helper cells using oligonucleotide arrays. Nat Genet 2000; 25(1):96-101.
14. Brazma A, Vilo J. Gene expression data analysis. FEBS Lett 2000; 480(1):17-24.
15. Eisen MB, Spellman PT, Brown PO et al. Cluster analysis and display of genome-wide expression patterns. Proc Natl Acad Sci USA 1998; 95(25):14863-8.
16. Nikkila J, Toronen P, Kaski S et al. Analysis and visualization of gene expression data using self-organizing maps. Neural Netw 2002; 15(8-9):953-66.
17. Crescenzi M, Giuliani A. The main biological determinants of tumor line taxonomy elucidated by a principal component analysis of microarray data. FEBS Lett 2001; 507(1):114-8.
18. Lin K, Kuang Y, Joseph JS et al. Conserved codon composition of ribosomal protein coding genes in Escherichia coli, Mycobacterium tuberculosis and Saccharomyces cerevisiae: Lessons from supervised machine learning in functional genomics. Nucleic Acids Res 2002; 30(11):2599-607.
19. Golub TR, Slonim DK, Tamayo P et al. Molecular classification of cancer: Class discovery and class prediction by gene expression monitoring. Science 1999; 286(5439):531-7.
20. Khan J, Wei JS, Ringner M et al. Classification and diagnostic prediction of cancers using gene expression profiling and artificial neural networks. Nat Med 2001; 7(6):673-9.
21. Alizadeh AA, Eisen MB, Davis RE et al. Distinct types of diffuse large B-cell lymphoma identified by gene expression profiling. Nature 2000; 403(6769):503-11.
22. Brown MP, Grundy WN, Lin D et al. Knowledge-based analysis of microarray gene expression data by using support vector machines. Proc Natl Acad Sci USA 2000; 97(1):262-7.
23. Mocellin S, Provenzano M, Rossi CR et al. DNA array-based gene profiling: From surgical specimen to the molecular portrait of Cancer. Ann Surg 2005; 241(1):16-26.

CHAPTER 4

Gaining Weights ... and Feeling Good about It!

Ernst Wit,* **Vilda Purutcuoglu, Lucy O'Donovan and Ximin Zhu**

Abstract

Two problems that dog current microarrays analyses are (i) the relatively arbitrary nature of data preprocessing and (ii) the inability to incorporate spot quality information in inference except by all-or-nothing spot filtering. In this chapter we propose an approach based on using weights to overcome these two problems. The first approach uses weighted p-values to make inference robust to normalization and the second approach uses weighted spot intensity values to improve inference without any filtering.

A Light Introduction

As with many other types of high-throughput technologies, microarray data require essential preprocessing steps in order to present it in a format that can be used for making inference. From the moment the actual experimental procedure have been completed after the hybridization a combination of several crucial steps have to be undertaken in order to get data. First of all the slides are scanned, which turns the number of attached mRNA molecules into collection of pixel values within an image. Then an image analysis package separates the background from the foreground signal (**gridding** and **segmentation**) and combines the pixel values into range of summaries (quantification). Those summaries typically consist of quantities like the mean, the median and the variance of the spot as well as the background pixel values. However, of those summaries, typically only a single value, namely the spot mean or median is used in inference. In section 3 we shall deal with ways we can use more of the available outputs in inference.

Those spot values are then frequently **normalized** across probe sets, array, channels or the whole experiment often changing the scale of the data via a number of possible algorithms, usually combined in some computer package (e.g., MAS 5.0, RMA, smida). This preprocessing of the physical, hybridized slides $S = (S_1, ..., S_s)$ into a data matrix of gene expression values $Y = (Y_1, ..., Y_s)$ can be represented via the action of the operator f

$$Y = f(S, v),$$

where, crucially, the v stands for all the parameters and normalization settings used in the preprocessing. In turn, these parameters are intended to capture the physical process of turning mRNA counts into an image into gene expression values. The precise value for v is typically unknown and depends highly on the skill of the technicians and software involved in the preprocessing steps for what seem **reasonable** choices. It is rare, although not impossible,

*Corresponding Author: Ernst Wit—Medical Statistics Unit, Department of Mathematics and Statistics, Lancaster University, Lancaster, LA1 1AE U.K. Email: e.wit@lancaster.ac.uk

Microarray Technology and Cancer Gene Profiling, edited by Simone Mocellin.
©2007 Landes Bioscience and Springer Science+Business Media.

that a value for v can be estimated from the data. Therefore, there is typically some level of arbitrariness in the choice of v. Slightly different values of v, e.g., v^*, will lead to different values of Y,

$$Y^* = f(S, v^*).$$

Which value should we actually use in our analysis? Y or Y^*, or perhaps some completely different Y^{**}. Most practical bioinformaticians would probably feel that they could live with this situation as long as they feel that they have made a "reasonable" choice for v. In that case, they would calculate, for example, their t-statistic $t_g(Y_g)$ for a particular gene g on the basis of the available data Y_g and calculate the two-sided p-value as

$$p - \text{value}(v) = 2p_{H_{0,v}}\left(T > \left|t_g(Y_g)\right|\right),$$

where H_0 is the null-hypothesis of no differential expression and, importantly, v the actually selected preprocessing parameters.

However, it is possible that different reasonable v-values will give rise to different answers, such as different significantly expressed genes—had one only tried. In section 2 we deal with the simple question to what extent we can accommodate the actual level of arbitrariness in the preprocessing of the data within our inference.

P-Value Weighting

If we have control over at least some of the nuisance parameters v, it is in principle possible to vary them to study their effects on inference. Consider for example that we could vary the gain settings on the scanner, the morphological properties of the image analysis programme or the parameters of the normalization procedures, which in total represents m different parameters, $v = (v_1, \ldots, v_m)$.

"Reasonable" values for v can be expressed as a hypothetical distribution on the parameters, p_v. This distribution expresses all the uncertainty about the preprocessing process—much in a way a Bayesian prior distribution would do. This uncertainty about v propagates into uncertainty about the data Y, which in turn modifies, for example, the p-value for gene g,

$$p - value(g) = P_{H_0}\left(T > \left|t_g(Y_g)\right|\right) = \int P_{H_{0,v}}\left(T > \left|t_g(Y_g)\right|\right)p_v(v)\partial v. \qquad (1)$$

This is the real p-value, i.e., the p-value that takes into account all the uncertainty about the data. In other words, the real p-value is a weighted average of all the naïve p-values at a particular normalization setting.

What does this mean in practice? As the normalization procedures can be extremely complex, it is unlikely that the integral in (1) can be solved explicitly. As a result, numeric integration via a discrete sum is the only way to make progress. In particular, if N = {$v^1, \ldots, v^k$} is the set of k normalization settings with weights $w_1, \ldots, w_k$, giving rise to k alternative data sets {$Y^1, \ldots, Y^k$}, then an approximate p-value can be calculated as

$$p - value(g) = \sum_{v \in N} w_v P_{0,v}\left(T > \left|t_g(Y_g)\right|\right) / \sum_{v \in N} w_v \qquad (2)$$

Effectively, the distribution $w_{v0}/\Sigma_v w_v$ is the discretised version the normalization parameter distribution. The true p-value is therefore a weighted sum of the p-values corresponding to the individual normalizations.

For good measure, we should add that in the presence of control spots on the microarray, the values of at least some of the preprocess parameters could be estimated directly from the data. This means that the subjective distribution pv can be replaced by an objective distribution, which now represents the uncertainty in the estimates of v. In case many of such control spots are present on the microarray and v can be estimated quite precisely, then inference can be done on the single normalized dataset where $v = \hat{v}$.

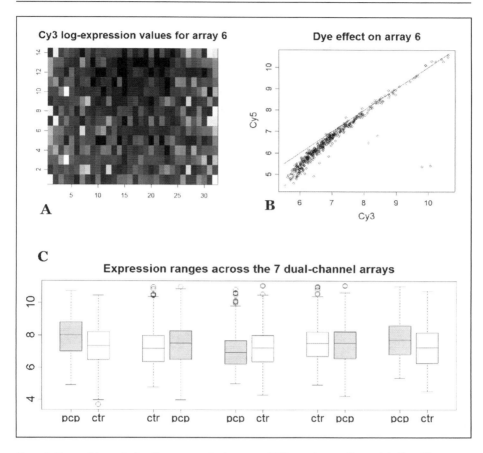

Figure 1. Some of the typical artifacts present in the mouse-PCP experiment: A) a spatial effect; B) a uneven dye effect; and C) a cross-comparison issue over the 7 arrays.

Application

Dr. Lucy O'Donovan (University of Glasgow) performed a microarray experiment, in which one of the aims was to find those genes that are differentially expressed in a mouse schizophrenia model as compared to in wild-type mice. The schizophrenia model was induced by treating the mice with a drug, PCP. Dr. O'Donovan hybridized the RNA from seven PCP and seven wild-type mice in a pairwise fashion to seven dual-channel microarrays. Each of the arrays contained 224 genes, spotted in duplicate. Although quality control measures suggested seven good hybridizations, with some transformation of the data several artifacts of the data were easy to spot by eye. In particular, there was some uneven hybridization across the arrays with darker areas in the top centre part of the array (Fig. 1A), some uneven dye effects (Fig. 1B) and also uneven gains between the arrays as evidenced by (Fig. 1C). In order to deal with these nuisance effects, we applied a series of preprocessing steps contained in the R-package smida. The mere default settings of the normalization procedures resulted in visually "improved" data (Figs. 2A-C).

The spatial normalization was done by fitting a first degree *loess* curve to both the mean and the standard deviation of the log-transformed data with span parameters equal to 0.5

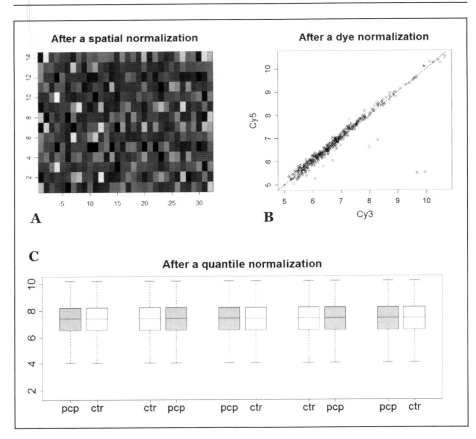

Figure 2. Preprocessing of the data helps to overcome: A) a spatial effect by brightening the top-centre part of the array; B) a uneven dye effect by boosting the Cy5 values in the lower expression ranges; and C) a cross-comparison issue by rescaling all the arrays to the same average distribution.

and 0.75 respectively. Changing the parameter values for the location normalization to 0.2 has no obvious visual effect on the normalization. We also consider a scale span parameter of 0.3 instead of 0.75.

By default the smida package does not subtract background, however settings are available to do either a probabilistic or deterministic background subtraction (details in ref. 1, sect. 4.3.3). The default setting for the *loess* dye normalization is a span of 0.2. By changing this span to 0.5 the adjustment becomes slightly less variable across the intensity range, although the effect is almost invisible. Similarly, for the quantile normalization one needs to specify a set of invariant genes. Complete quantile normalization implicitly assumes that all genes are invariant. We also considered invariant set sizes of 30 and 100 genes out of all 224 genes. Taken altogether, we considered

2 spat loc × 2 spat scale × 3 bkg × 2 dye × 3 quantile = 72 normalizations

Each of these normalizations resulted in an alternative normalized dataset. In each of these datasets, we could proceed to test for differential expression across each of the 224 genes. Standard normal quantile plots suggest that the normal assumption is not inappropriate and that therefore a t-test can be used to find differences between PCP and control mice.

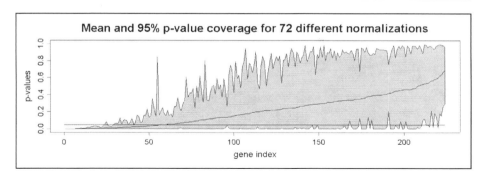

Figure 3. For each of the 72 normalizations and for each of the 224 genes we calculate all of the p-values for testing for differential expression between PCR and control mice. For each of the genes, we indicate the range between the 3rd smallest and 70th largest p-value (approx. 95% coverage), as well as the average p-value.

Figure 3 shows the range of p-values across 72 normalizations for the 224 genes. The genes are arbitrarily ordered by an increasing average p-value, indicated by the solid line in Figure 3. First of all, it is striking to see the impact of the preprocessing on the actual inference from the data.

As we a priori do not have any information to suggest which of the normalizations is better, we regard each of the 72 parameter settings as equally plausible, i.e., $p_V(v) = 1/72$. Consequently, the p-value that is robust to preprocessing is simply given as the average p-value across all 72 normalizations. From Figure 3, we see that 23 genes have a p-value less than 0.01, 59 genes have a p-value less than 0.05. If we use the Benjamini and Hochberg[2] procedure, we find 88 genes that such that the false discovery rate is less than 5%. Clearly, if there had been any control spots on the array for which we could get some idea of the relative plausibility of the normalization parameters, then the relative weights and therefore the resulting p-value would change. Nevertheless, inference based on the average p-value based on several normalizations has the distinct advantage of making inference less susceptible to some arbitrary settings.

Within-Spot Pixel Variance Weighting

That not every gene expression measurement is as good as another is well known in the microarray community. Soon after the introduction of microarrays, imaging programmes introduced the idea of spot filtering: a method whereby unreliable spots were flagged in order to remove them from analysis. Even in its crudest form, flagging is an example of 0-1 weighting. However, there is no reason why these all-or-nothing weights cannot be replaced by more realistic, continuous weights. In this section, we derive a simple method for introducing continuous weights.

In this section we assume that the quality of a spot can be indicated by means of a single value, which corresponds to the within-spot pixel standard deviation. Highly variable spots have a large within-spot pixel standard deviation, whereas good quality, homogeneous spots have small within-spot pixel standard deviations.

Let x_i stand for the ith spot intensity, associated with one particular gene. If we have n spots associated with the same gene, then we can write the spot standard deviations as proportional to the within-spot pixel standard deviation,

$$SD(x_i) \propto \sigma_i, \qquad i = 1,\ldots,n$$

where the constant of proportionality depends on the number of pixels in a spot, the spatial correlation between the spot pixels, which we assume constant across different spots.

If the aim of the experiment is to estimate the true mean expression μ for that particular gene as accurate as possible, then the best estimate can be written as a weighted mean of all the observed expression values,

$$\hat{\mu} = \sum_{i=1}^{n} w_i x_i.$$

If none of the expression values displays any particular bias, then in order for the estimate to be unbiased, the weights should add up to one, $\sum_{i=1}^{n} w_i = 1$. In order to minimize the variance of the estimate, $V(\hat{\mu}) \propto \sum_{i=1}^{n} w_i^2 \sigma_i^2$, it is easy to show that the optimal choice of weights should be proportional to the inverse of the pixel variance in each of the spots,

$$w_i = \frac{1/\sigma_i^2}{\sum_{k=1}^{n} 1/\sigma_k^2}. \tag{3}$$

Although weighting with the within-spot pixel standard deviation is a good idea, there are a few issues that remain to be solved: (i) as the within-spot pixel standard deviations are not known, they have to be estimated from the data; (ii) if the analysis is done on the logarithmic scale, then an appropriate estimate of the within-spot log pixel variance needs to be produced.

Dealing with an Unknown within-Spot Pixel Variance

In order to use the weighting formula in equation (3), we need to replace the unknown within-spot pixel variance with some estimate thereof. The typical output of an imaging and segmentation programme will provide an estimate of the within-spot variance, $\hat{\tau}_i^2$. As we can expect a large amount of spatial correlation between neighbouring pixels, it is likely that this quantity is a severe underestimate of the within-spot pixel variance. Nevertheless, this affects each spot more or less equally and therefore the approximately multiplicative constant should disappear from equation (3).

The most straightforward thing to do would be to replace the within-spot pixel variance σ_i^2 with the estimated within-spot variance $\hat{\tau}_i^2$ in equation (3). However, there may be good reasons to consider a slightly more general approach, namely:

$$\sigma_i^2 \longleftarrow \hat{\tau}_i^2 + a. \tag{4}$$

Taking $a = 0$ is equivalent to using the within-spot variance, whereas if $a \to \infty$ then this would correspond to an unweighted or simple average approach. The reason why adding a constant may have some benefit is that the estimated within-spot variance is itself subject to variation and this constant would robustify the weighting somewhat.

Bakewell and Wit[3] propose a biologically motivated choice for the constant a by replacing it with the estimate of the inherent biological variation for any sample—or in statistical terms, the **subject effect**. Other, more ad hoc choices for a can include some quantile of the observed within-spot variances $\hat{\tau}_i^2$; the higher the quantile, the more conservative and robust the estimate of the weighted mean.

Analysis of the Data on a Log Transformed Scale

Some people prefer to do the analysis microarray data on the logarithmic scale.[4,5] The reason is that the spot intensities are per definition positive, so that it is quite likely that any dominant effects will be multiplicative, rather than additive. Log transforming multiplicative effects will transform the data to an additive scale, which makes analysis more straightforward.

However, most summary information from imaging files is—still—provided on the original pixel scale. Although it would be very useful to have information such as the mean and variance of the log pixel spot values, such information is typically not available. Something can be done, however, in the absence of such information. As is already common, instead of the mean of the log of the spot pixel values, one can use the log of the mean of those values. In order to get some approximation of the variance of the log pixel values, we can consider the following first order Taylor approximation around the spot mean,

$$V\left(\log(X)\right) \approx V\left(EX + (X - EX)\frac{1}{EX}\right) = \frac{V(X)}{E^2(X)}.$$

This equality means that we can approximate the variance of the log pixel values by the original spot pixel variance divided by the square of the original spot pixel mean. An easy way to proceed, therefore, would be as follows:

1. Take as expression values $x_1, ..., x_n$,

   $x_i = log\ spot\ mean$

2. Take as robust expression variances $s_1^2, ..., s_n^2$,

   $s_i^2 = spot\ variance/(spot\ mean)^2 + a$

3. Take as weights $w_1, ..., w_n$,

$$w_i = \frac{1/s_i^2}{\sum_{k=1}^{n} 1/s_k^2}.$$

4. Calculate the average expression as

$$\hat{\mu} = \sum_{i=1}^{n} w_i x_i.$$

This estimate of the true of expression μ can then be used for further inference, for example, in a test for differential expression. Unfortunately, normal theory does not apply to weighted means, especially for few replicates. Alternatives, such as bootstrap and permutation tests are however directly applicable.

A Weighty Discussion

Preprocessing the data can have a substantial impact on further inference. It is a mistake to assume that the preprocessed data is a unique abstraction of the actual dataset, uniquely suitable for inference. In fact, preprocessing is itself a form of data analysis, which carries along with it all the uncertainty of choosing the correct settings for the normalization parameters. We presented **p-value weighting** as a method to overcome some of the trouble of basing one's conclusions on a single preprocessed dataset.

The method has two main drawbacks. First of all, it requires substantial computational efforts to generate a large number of preprocessed datasets on which to perform the same analysis. As all of the computations are completely parallel, there may be some gain in using parallel computing facilities to overcome some of the computational effort. Even if the computational issue can be overcome, the method is only applicable to hypothesis testing. Only p-values can be "averaged out" over the different datasets, whereas estimates, clusterings or predictions cannot. Nevertheless, the idea of applying the same analysis technique, be it clustering, prediction or something else, to different preprocessed datasets can certainly provide valuable insights. If a particular clustering is stable under the vast majority of all the possible normalizations, then this will strengthen our confidence in the conclusions.

The idea of **spot pixel variance weighting** is sensible because it uses more of the information available in the data, which should lead to better answers. In this sense weighting is similar to data filtering methods. However, spot weighting avoids getting missing values, which is a drawback of most filtering methods.

Should spot weighting be used everywhere? In general, the answer is *yes*. There is valuable information in the output of most imaging and segmentation software. Ignoring such information is equivalent with habitually throwing away a few arrays. Even in cases where the spot pixel variances are slightly suspect or based on only a small number of pixels, combining the observed values with a robustifying choice of constant a is expected to improve inference.

Nevertheless, there are a few cases in which using spot pixel variance might be inappropriate: (i) if the quality of a spot is seriously affected by things others than measured in the spot variance; (ii) if the physical meaning of the spot variance changes between arrays. An example of the former is the quality of the RNA used for hybridizing different arrays or the presence of smears and stains, which all may have no influence on the spot variance as such, but does affect the quality of an individual measurement. An example of the latter is a large difference in the gain or large differences in the number of pixels used for spots between different arrays.

References

1. Wit E, McClure JD. Statistics for microarrays: Design, analysis and inference. Chichester: J Wiley and Sons, 2004.
2. Benjamini Y, Hochberg Y. Controlling the false discovery rate: A practical and powerful approach to multiple testing. J Royal Statistical Society B 1995; 57:289-300.
3. Bakewell D, Wit E. Weighted analysis of microarray gene expression using maximum-likelihood. Bioinformatics 2005; 21(6):723-9.
4. Irizarry RA, Gautier L, Cope LM. An R package for analyses of Affymetrix oligonucleotide arrays. In: Parmigiani G, Garrett ES, Irizarry RA, eds. The Analysis of Gene Expression Data. Statistics for Biology and Health. New York: Springer-Verlag, 2003:102-19.
5. Kerr M, Churchill GA. Experimental design for gene expression microarrays. Biostatistics 2001; (2):183-201.

CHAPTER 5.1

Complementary Techniques:
RNA Amplification for Gene Profiling Analysis

Ena Wang, Monica Panelli, and Francesco M. Marincola*

Abstract

The study of clinical samples is often limited by the amount of material available. DNA and RNA can be amplified from small specimens and, therefore, used for high-throughput analyses. While precise estimates of the level of DNA concentration in a given specimen is rarely studied (with the exception of relatively crude analyses of gene amplification or loss in cancer specimens), it is critical to know the proportional expression of various RNA transcripts since this proportion governs cell function by modulating the expression of various proteins. In addition, accurate estimates of relative RNA expression in biological conditions portray the reaction of cells to environmental stimuli shedding light on the characteristics of the microenvironment associated with particular physiologic or pathologic conditions. For this reason, the development of technologies for high fidelity messenger RNA amplification have been focused of extreme interest in the past decade with specific aim not only of increasing the abundance of RNA available to study but to accurately maintain the proportionality of expression of various RNA species among each other within a given specimen. This chapter will discuss various approaches to proportional RNA amplification focusing on amplification of the whole transcriptome (all transcripts in a given samples) rather than individual genes. These methods are suitable for high-throughput transcriptional profiling studies.

Introduction

Quantification of gene expression has become a very powerful tool in understanding the molecular biology underlying complex pathophysiological conditions. Advances in gene profiling analysis using cDNA or oligo-based microarray systems uncovered genes critically important in disease development, progression, and response to treatment.[1-12] While the expression of a single or a limited number of genes can be readily estimated using minimum amount of total or messenger RNA (mRNA) obtained from experimental or clinic samples, gene profiling requires large amounts of RNA, which can only be generated from RNA amplification, particularly in the case of biological material obtained from humans. At least 50-100 μg of total RNA (T-RNA) or 2-5 μg poly(A)+ RNA are generally necessary for gene profiling experiments which can only be generated from cultured cell lines or large excisional biopsies.[13] However, most biological specimens directly obtained ex vivo for diagnostic or prognostic purposes or for clinic monitoring during treatment are too scarce to yield enough RNA for high-throughput gene expression analysis. Fine needle aspirates or punch biopsies

*Corresponding Author: Francesco M. Marincola—Department of Transfusion Medicine, Clinical Center, National Institutes of Health, Immunogenetics Section, 9000 Rockville Pike Bethesda, Maryland 20892 U.S.A. Email: FMarincola@cc.nih.gov

Microarray Technology and Cancer Gene Profiling, edited by Simone Mocellin.
©2007 Landes Bioscience and Springer Science+Business Media.

provide the opportunity to serially sample lesions during treatment or sample before treatment to follow the treatment outcome of the lesion left in place. In addition, the simplicity of the storage procedure associated with the collection of small samples provides superior quality of RNA with minimum degradation.[14] Finally, the hypoxia that follows ligation of tumor-feeding vessels before excision is avoided with these minimally invasive methods therefore obtaining a true snapshot of the in vivo transcriptional program. However, these minimally invasive biopsies can yield few micrograms and most often less total RNA.[14,15] Similarly, breast and nasal lavages and cervical brush biopsies, routinely used in pathological diagnosis, generate insufficient material far below the fluorescent labeling detection. Acquisition of cell subsets by fluorescent or magnetic sorting or laser capture microdissection (LCM) for a more accurate portraying of individual cell interactions in a pathological process generate even less material, in most cases, nano grams of total RNA.[16-19]

Efforts have been made to broaden the utilization of cDNA microarrays using two main strategies: intensifying fluorescence signal[20-23] or amplifying RNA. Signal intensification approaches have reduced the requirement of RNA few folds but cannot extend the utilization of microarray to sub-microgram RNA quantities. RNA amplification in turn has gained extreme popularity based on amplification efficiency, linearity and reproducibility lowering the amount of total RNA needed for microarray analysis to nanograms without introducing significant biases. Methods aimed at the amplification of poly(A)-RNA[24] via in vitro transcription (IVT)[25] or cDNA amplification via polymerase chain reaction (PCR)[26] have reduced the material needed for cDNA microarray application and extended the spectrum of clinic samples that can be studied. Nanograms of total RNA have been successfully amplified into micrograms of pure mRNA for the screening of the entire transcriptome without losing the proportionality of gene expression displayed by the source material. Modifications, optimizations and validations of RNA amplification technology based on Eberwine's pioneering work are still actively explored.

In this chapter, we will summarize efforts to optimize RNA amplification and describe in detail current amplification procedures that have been validated and applied to cDNA microarray analysis.

Source Material Collection and RNA Isolation

Samples used for RNA isolation and amplification should always be collected fresh and immediately processed. Excisional biopsies should be handled within 20 min and stored at -80°C with RNAlater™ (Ambion, Cat# 7020) if isolation cannot be performed right away. Material from fine needle aspirates (FNA) should be put in 5 ml of ice-cold 1x PBS or other collection medium without serum at the patient's bedside to minimize RNA metabolism or degradation. After spinning at 1,500 rpm for 5 min at 4°C, add 2.5 ml of ACK lysing buffer with 2.5 ml of 1x PBS and incubate for 5 min on ice to lyse red blood cells (RBC) in case of excessive contamination. Cell pellet should be washed in 10 ml 1x PBS and then resuspend in small volume of RNA later followed by snap freeze or lyse pellet in 350 μl of RLT buffer with fresh addition of 2-mercaptoethanol (2-ME) according to manufacture's manual (RNeasy mini kit, QIAGEN Inc, Valencia, CA, USA) and then snap freeze at -80°C. For laser capture micro-dissected (LCM) samples, good results can be obtained by lysing cells directly in 50 μl RLT buffer with 2-ME per cap and snap freeze at -80°C. Total RNA and poly-A RNA can both be used as starting material for RNA amplification.

The RNA isolation method strongly affects the quality and quantity of RNA. Total RNA (T-RNA) can be isolated using commercially available RNA isolation kits by following the manufacturer's instructions. The total RNA content per mammalian cell is in the range of 20-40 pg of which only 0.5-1.0 pg are constituted by mRNA.[27,28] Sample condition, viability, functional status and phenotype of the cells are the major reasons for differential yield of T-RNA. Sample handling with precaution for RNase contamination always improves the quality and quantity of the RNA obtained. Measurement of T-RNA concentration can be performed with a spectrophotometer at OD_{260}. An $OD_{260/280}$ ratio above 1.8 is to be expected. When a very limited number of cells is available such as from LCM or FNA, very low or even negative OD readings may be observed. In this case, OD reading can be omitted. When RNA is isolated from archive samples or from samples whose collection and storage conditions were not controlled and optimized, it is preferable to estimate RNA quality and quantity using Agilent Bioanalyzer or RNA gels. Clear 28S and 18S ribosomal RNA bands indicate good quality of RNA. Since 28S rRNA degradation occurs earlier than 18S and mRNA degradation in most cases correlates with 28S ribosomal RNA, the ratio of 28S versus 18S rRNA is a good indicator of mRNA quality.[29] 28S/18S rRNA ratios equal or close to 2 suggest good RNA quality.

Single-Strand cDNA Synthesis

A critical step in RNA or cDNA amplification is the generation of double-stranded cDNA (ds-cDNA) templates. First-strand cDNAs are reverse transcribed from mRNA using oligo-dT or random primers. In order to generate full length first-strand cDNA, oligo-dT (15-24 nt) with an attachment of a bacterial phage T7 promoter sequence is commonly used to initiate the cDNA synthesis.[24,30-34] In case of degraded RNA,[35] random primers with attachment of T3 RNA polymerase promoter (T3N9) have been used for first and second-strand cDNA synthesis.[36] To prevent RNA degradation while denaturing and during the reverse transcription RT reaction, it is useful to denature the RNA (65°C for 5 min or 70°C for 3 min) in the presence of RNasin® Plus RNase Inhibitor (Promega) which forms a stable complex with RNases and inactivates RNase at temperatures up to 70°C for at least 15 min.

To enhance the efficiency of the RT reaction and reduce incorporation errors, the temperature of the RT reaction can be maintained at 50°C[37,38] instead of 42°C to avoid the formation of secondary mRNA structures. This can be attained by using thermostable reverse transcriptase (ThermoScript™ RNase-H Reverse Transcriptase) (Invitrogen; cat# 12236022) or regular RTase[39] in the presence of disaccharide trehalose.[40-42] Disaccharide trehalose not only can enhance the thermostability of RTase but also has thermoactivation function to the enzyme. This modification greatly enhances the accuracy and the efficiency of RT reactions, with minimum impact on the DNA polymerase activity of RTase.[37] The utilization of DNA binding protein T4gp32 (USB, Cleveland; 400 ng/µl) in RT reaction has also been shown to enhance PCR and cDNA synthesis.[38,39,43,44] T4gp32 protein may essentially contribute to the qualitative and quantitative efficiency of the RT reaction by reducing higher order structure of RNA molecules and hence reduce the pause sites during cDNA synthesis.

In Van Gelder and Eberwine's T7-based RNA amplification,[45] the amount of oligo-dT-T7 primer used in the first-strand cDNA synthesis can affect the amplified RNA in quantity and quality. Excessive oligo-dT-T7 in the RT reaction could lead to template independent amplification.[46] This phenomenon is not observed when the template switch approach is used in in vitro transcription.

Double-Stranded cDNA (ds-cDNA) Synthesis

RNA amplification methods differ according to the strategies used for the generation of ds-cDNA as templates for in vitro transcription or PCR amplification. There are two basic strategies that have been extensive validated and applied for high-throughput transcriptional analysis. The first is based on Gubler-Hoffman's[47] ds-cDNA synthesis subsequently optimized by Van Gelder and Eberwine.[30,45] This technology utilizes RNase H digestion to create short fragments of RNA as primers to initiate the second-strand cDNA elongation under DNA polymerase-I. Fragments of second-strand cDNA are then ligated to each other sequentially under *E. coli* DNA ligase followed by polishment using T4 DNA polymerase to eliminate loops and to form blunt ends. Amplifications based on this methods has been widely used in samples obtained in physiological or pathological conditions and extensively validated for its fidelity, reproducibility and linearity compared to un-amplified RNA from the same source materials.[30,31,46,48-51]

The alternative ds-cDNA synthesis approach utilizes retroviral RNA recombination as a mechanism for template switch to generate full-length ds-cDNA. The method was initially invented for full-length cDNA cloning and, therefore, the main targets of this method are undegredated transcripts. Gubler-Hoffman's ds-cDNA synthesis has the potential of introducing amplification biases because of a possible 5' under-representation. In addition, the low stringency of the temperature in which ds-cDNA synthesis occurs may introduce additional biases.[31] Although 5' under-representation could, in theory, be overcome by hairpin loop second-strand synthesis,[52] the multiple enzymes (4) used in the reaction could also in turn cause errors.

To ensure generation of full-length ds-cDNA,[53] synthesis is performed taking advantage of the intrinsic terminal transferase activity and template switch ability of Moloney Murine Leukemia Virus (MMLV) reverse transcriptase (RTase).[54] This enzyme adds nontemplate nucleotides at the 3'-end of the first-strand cDNA, preferentially dCTP oligo nucleotides. A template-switch oligonucleotide (TS primer) containing a short string of dG residues at the 3'-end is added to the reaction to anneal to the dC string of the newly synthesized cDNA. This produces an overhang that allows the RTase to switch template and extend the cDNA beyond the dC to create a short segment of double stranded cDNA duplex. After treatment with RNase H to remove the original mRNA, the TS primer initiates the second-stranded cDNA synthesis under polymerase chain reaction (PCR). Since the terminal transferase activity of the RTase is triggered only when the cDNA synthesis is complete, only full-length single stranded cDNA will be tailed with the TS primer and converted into ds-cDNA. Using the TS primer, second-strand cDNA synthesis is carried at 75°C after a 95°C denaturing and a 65°C annealing step in the presence of single DNA polymerase.[33] This technique, in theory, overcomes the bias generated by amplification methods depending only on 3'-nucleotide synthesis and hence it is, in theory, superior to the Gubler-Hoffman's ds-cDNA synthesis. However, no significant differences in correlation coefficients of amplified versus non amplified RNA were observed when the Gubler-Hoffman's ds-cDNA method was compared with the TS ds-cDNA amplification using high-throughput analysis.[38,55] The fidelity of template switch-based amplification method has been assessed by numerous gene profiling analyses on different type of microarray platforms, real time PCR and sophisticated statistical analyses and it has been well accepted for high-throughput transcriptome studies.

RNA Amplification

Linear Amplification

Amplifying populations of mRNAs without skewing their relative abundances remains a hot focus of research interest. Linear amplification methods have been developed that in theory should maintain the proportionality of each RNA species present in the original sample. In vitro transcription (IVT) using ds-cDNA equipped with a bacteriophage T7 promoter[45] provides an efficient way to amplify mRNA sequences and thereby generate templates for synthesis of fluorescently-labeled single-stranded cDNA.[24,25,30,31,45,52] Depending upon the T7 or other (T3 or SP6) promoter sequence position on the ds-cDNA, amplified RNA can be either in sense or antisense orientation. Oligo-dT attachments to the promoter sequence, for example oligo-dT-T7, prime first-strand cDNA at the 3'-end of genes (5'-end of cDNA) and, therefore, lead to the amplification of antisense RNA (aRNA) or complement RNA (cRNA). Promoters positioned at the 5'-end of genes (3' end of the cDNA) by random[56] or TS primers generate sense RNA (sRNA). Amplified sRNA can be also produced by tailing of oligo-dT to the 3' of the cDNA followed by oligo-dA-T7 priming for double-stranded T7 promoter generation at the 5'-end of genes.[57] The singularity of this approach resides in the utilization of a DNA polymerase blocker at the 3' of the oligo-dA-T7 primer, which prevents the elongation of second-strand cDNA synthesis while priming for the elongation of the double stranded promoter. In this fashion, only sense amplification can be achieved by the presence of the 5' double strand T7 promoter followed by single strand cDNA templates.

IVT using DNA-dependent RNA polymerase is an isothermal reaction with linear kinetics. The input ds-cDNA templates are the only source of template for the complete amplification and therefore, any errors created on the newly synthesized RNA will not be carried or amplified in the following reactions. Overall, RNA polymerase makes an error at a frequency of about once in 10,000 nucleotides corresponding to about once per RNA strand created (http://www.rcsb.org/pdb/molecules/pdb40_1.html). This contrasts with DNA-dependent DNA polymerase, which incorporates an error once in every 400 nucleotides. Most importantly, these errors are exponentially amplified in the following reaction since the amplicons serve as templates. In spite of the lower error rate, RNA polymerase catalyzes transcription robotically and efficiently without sequence dependent bias. Recombinant RNA polymerases have been engineered to enhance the stability of the enzyme interacting with templates and reduce the abortive tendency[58] of the wild type RNA polymerase, which in turn improved the elongation phase resulting in complete mRNA transcripts. The length of amplified RNA ranges from 200 to 6,000 nucleotides for the first round of amplification and 100 to 3,000 nucleotides for the second round when random primers are used.[34,59] The amplification efficiency is greater than 2,000 folds in the first round and 100,000 folds in the second round.[33,59]

Two rounds of IVT are commonly required when sub micrograms of input total RNA are used (Fig. 1). It has been estimated that after two rounds amplification the frequency of about 10% of genes is reduced[60] and more than two rounds of amplification may still retain at least in part the proportionality of gene expression among different RNA populations.[33] However, we do not recommend going over two rounds of amplification unless necessary when processing single or few cell specimens, to avoid unnecessary biases related to amplification. The fidelity of IVT has been extensively assessed by gene profiling analysis, quantitative real-time PCR and statistical testing by comparing estimates of gene expression in amplified versus nonamplified RNA.[33]

Pitfalls have been also associated with IVT. The fidelity of the first-round amplification decreases when the input starting material is less than 100 ng because of the intrinsic low abundance of transcripts (particularly those under represented in the biological specimen). This can be rescued by two rounds of IVT if sufficient RNA species are present in the input material.[33] In addition, two rounds of amplification tend to introduce a 3' bias due to the usage of random primer in the cDNA synthesis for ds-cDNA template creation. This should not affect the usefulness of the technique for the of transcript for high-throughput gene profiling analysis since cloned cDNA arrays are 3'-biased and even oligo-arrays are designed to target the 3'-end of each gene. Sequence-specific biases introduced during amplification are generally reproducible and, although negligible, could mislead data interpretation only when amplified RNA is directly compared with nonamplified RNA on the same array platform. This type of error can be easily circumvented by using samples processed in identical conditions. Degradation of amplified RNA during prolonged (more than 5 hours) IVT may result in lower average size of RNA and decreased yields.[35] This results from residual RNase in the enzyme mixture used for IVT reaction and can be prevented by the addition of RNase inhibitor in the reaction, if a prolonged amplification is needed.

PCR-Based Exponential Amplification

The drawbacks of linear amplification (IVT) are time consuming and the possible 3'-bias, especially when two rounds of amplification are employed. Exponential amplification (PCR-based) on the other hand, has shown promise and has recently attracted attention. This approach, contrary to the IVT, is simple and efficient.

The limitations of PCR-based amplification stem from the characteristics of the DNA-dependent DNA polymerase enzymatic function. The function of this enzyme is biased towards a lower efficiency in the amplification of GC rich sequences compared with AT rich sequences. In addition, as previously discussed, not only creates errors more frequently than RNA polymerase but also amplifies these mistakes because the reaction utilizes the amplicons

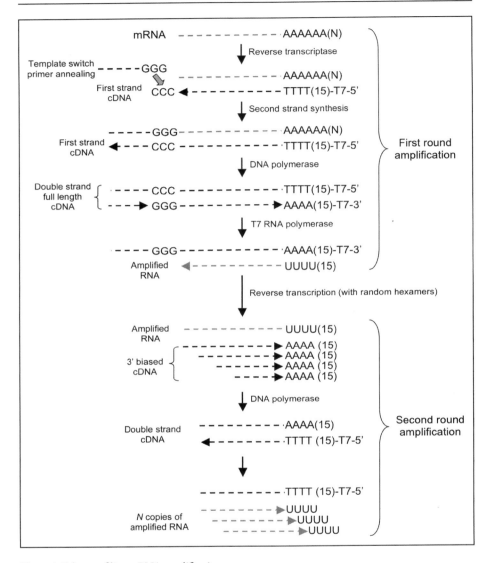

Figure 1. Scheme of linear RNA amplification.

as templates for subsequent amplification.[61] In addition, due to the exponential amplification, the reaction could reach saturation in conditions of excess input template used or because of the exhaustion of substrate. This would favor the amplification of high-abundance transcripts, which would compete more efficiently for substrate in the earlier cycles of the amplification process resulting in loss of linearity of the amplification process. Optimization in PCR cycle number to avoid reaching the saturation cycle and adjustments in the amount of template input could overcome the problems.[62] The utilization of DNA polymerase with proofreading function could eradicate errors created in the cDNA amplification.[63] This approach preserves the relative abundance transcript[64] and it may outperform IVT when less than 50 ng of input RNA are available as starting material.[65,66]

PCR-based cDNA amplification can be categorized as template switching (TS)-PCR,[51,67,68] random PCR[69] and 3' tailing with 5' adaptor ligation PCR[70] based on the generation of a 5' anchor sequence which provides a platform for 5' primer annealing. TS-PCR employs the same template switch mechanism in ds-cDNA generation and in the amplification of ds-cDNA using 5' TS primer II (truncated TS primer) and 3' oligo-dT or dT-T7 primers (depending upon the primer used in the first-strand cDNA synthesis). Random PCR utilizes modified oligo-dT primers (dT-T7 or dT-TAS [Target Amplification Sequence]) or random primers with an adaptor sequence for the first-strand cDNA initiation and random primers with an attachment of the same adaptor, for example dN10-TAS,[69] for second-strand cDNA synthesis. The attached sequence, such as TAS, generates a 5'-anchor on the cDNA for subsequent PCR amplification with a single TAS-PCR primer. This approach is more suitable for RNA with partial degradation and with the risk of under representation of the 5'-end. The third exponential amplification utilizes terminal deoxynucleotidyl transferase function to add a polymonomer tail (e.g., poly-dA) to the 5'-end of the gene. The tailed poly-dA provides an annealing position for the oligo-dT primer, which leads the second-strand cDNA synthesis. Double-stranded cDNA can then be amplified under one oligo-dT primer or dT-adaptor primer if an adaptor sequence is attached.[65] Direct adaptor ligation is another alternative way to generate ds-cDNA with a known anchor sequence at the 5'-end.[70] In this way, single strand cDNA is generated using oligo-dT primers immobilized onto magnetic beads and second-strand cDNA is completed by Van Gelder and Eberwine's ds-cDNA generation method. A ds-T7 promoter-linker is then unidirectionally ligated to the blunted ds-cDNA at the 5'-end. PCR amplification can then be performed using the 5' promoter primer and the 3' oligo-dT or dT-adapter primer, if an adapter is attached. PCR amplified ds-cDNA is suitable for either sense or antisense probe arrays.

The combination of PCR amplification to generate sufficient ds-cDNA template followed by IVT[69,70] is an attractive strategy to amplify minimal starting material since it takes advantage of the efficiency of the PCR reaction and the linear kinetics of IVT while minimizing the disadvantage discussed above. Validations of PCR-based RNA amplification methods are fewer than those for IVT but have been so far persuasive in spite of the prevalent expectations. Skepticism concerning the reproducibility and linearity are still one of the key factors preventing the extensive application of this approach. Protocols and procedures using PCR-based amplification—which has not achieved much success among researchers—will not be discussed further in the current chapter.

Target Labeling for cDNA Microarray Using Amplified RNA

The generation of high quality cDNA microarray data depends not only on sufficient amount and highly representative amplified target, but also on the target labeling efficacy and reproducibility. Steps involved in the targets preparation such as RNA amplification, target labeling, prehybridization, hybridization and slides washing are imperative in enhancing foreground signal to background noise ratios. Linear spectrum of signal intensity that correlates with gene copy numbers without having to compensate detection sensitivity is one of the key factors for high quality cDNA analysis. Therefore, target labeling is a critical step to achieve consistently high signal images.

Typically, fluorescently-labeled cDNA is generated by incorporation of conjugated nucleotide analogs during the reverse transcription process. Depending upon the detection system, labeled markers can be either radioactive, color matrix or florescent. Florescence labeling outperforms the other labeling methods because of the versatile excitation and emission wave length. In addition, it has the advantage of not being hazardous. Among fluorochromes, Cy3 (N,N8-(dipropyl)-tetramethylindocarbocyanine) and Cy5 (N,N8-(dipropyl)-tetramethylindodicarbocyanine) are most commonly used in cDNA microarray applications due to their distinct emission (510 and 664 respectively). Cy5-labeled dUTP and dCTP are less efficient in incorporation during the labeling reaction compared to Cy3-labeled dUTP or dCTP and they are more sensitive to photo bleach because of their chemical structure. Therefore, labeling bias needs to be accurately analyzed and results should be normalized according to standard normalization procedures.

Target labeling can be divided into two major categories: direct fluorescence incorporation and indirect fluorescence incorporation (see chapter on target preparation and labeling). The first category utilizes fluorescence-labeled dUTP or dCTP to partially substitute unlabeled dTTP or dCTP in the RT reaction to generate Cydye-labeled cDNA. This label incorporation method is suitable for cDNA clone microarray using amplified aRNA as templates or oligo array using amplified sRNA as template. In order to generate labeled aRNA target, which could hybridize to sense oligo array, direct labeling of aRNA is performed in the IVT reaction with biotin or Dig labeled CTP or UTP (Affymetrix standard protocol). The problem with this approach is the easily detachment of the RNA polymerase from the template when modified NTP are incorporated resulting in the premature termination of the elongation reaction.

A limitation of direct labeling consists in the fact that fluorescent nucleotides are not the normal substrates for polymerases and some may be particularly sensitive to the structural diversity of these artificial oligonucleotides. The fluorescent moieties associated with these nucleotides are often quite bulky and, therefore, the efficiency of incorporation of such nucleotides by polymerase tends to be much lower than that of natural substrates. An alternative is to incorporate, either by synthesis or by enzymatic activity, a nucleotide analog similar to the natural nucleotide in structure featuring a chemically reactive group, such as 5-(3-Aminoallyl)-2'-deoxyuridine 5'-triphosphate (aa-dUTP), to which a fluorescent dye, such as Cydye, may then be attached.[71] The reactive amine of the aa-dUTP can be incorporated by a variety of RNA-dependent and DNA-dependent DNA polymerases. After removing free nucleotides, the aminoallyl-labeled samples can coupled to dye, purified again, and then applied to a microarray.[72] The optimized ratio of aa-dUTP versus dTTP in the labeling reaction should be 2 to 3 respectively.

In theory, indirect outperforms direct labeling by reducing of the cost and maximizing signal intensity through increases in incorporation of fluorochrome or through signal amplification using fluorescence-labeled antibody or biotin-streptavidin complexes. However, more steps are involved in the purification of the labeled target prior to hybridization, which makes this strategies less frequently used.

Appendix: RNA Amplification Protocol

In this section, only the TS-IVT and Eberwine's RNA amplification protocols will be described in detail.

Materials and Reagents

The following is the list of reagents needed for RNA amplification. Enzymes, primers and columns are listed separately. Dilute stock solution to the appropriate working concentration.

- 5x first-strand buffer (comes with Superscript-II enzyme)
- 10x second-strand buffer (Invitrogen; cat#10812-014)
- dNTP mix solution (dATP, dCTP, dGTP, dTTP, 10 mM each) (Pharmacia; cat#27-2035-02)
- Low-T dNTP (5 mM dA, dG and dCTP, 2 mM dTTP)
- 0.1 M DTT (Dithioerythritol, molecular biology grade)
- RNasin Plus (20 units/μl) (Promega cat#N2611)
- Advantage PCR buffer (come with Advantage cDNA polymerase)
- Linear Acrylamide (0.1 μg/μl. Ambion; cat#9520)
- Phenol: Chloroform: Isoamyl alcohol (25:24:1) (Boehringer Mannhem cat#101001)
- Phase Lock gel (heavy) (5 prime to 3 prime, Inc.; cat#pl-188233)
- 7.5 M ammonium acetate (Sigma; cat#A2706)
- DEPC treated H_2O
- 75 mM NTP (A, G, C and UTP) (come with IVT kit)
- In Vitro Tanscription Kit (Ambion; T7 Megascript Kit #1334)

- Cy-dUTP (1 mM Cy3 or Cy5) (Ameishan Life Science)
- 1 M NaOH
- 500 mM EDTA
- 1x TE
- 1 M Tris pH 7.5
- 50x Denhardt's blocking solution (Sigma; cat# 2532)
- Poly-dA$_{40\text{-}60}$ (8 µg/µl) (Pharmacia; cat# 27-7988-01)
- Human Cot-I DNA (10 µg/µl) (Invitrogen; cat# 15279-011)
- 20x SSC
- 10% SDS
- ACK lysing buffer
- T4gp32 protein (8 µg/µl) (USB; cat# 74029Y)

Enzymes
- RNase HMMLV Reverse Transcriptase (200 U/µl) (Invitrogen; cat#18064-071)
- 50x Advantage cDNA polymerase mix (Clontech; cat#8417-1)
- RNase-H (2 U/µl, Invitrogen; cat#18021-071)
- *E. coli* DNA polymerase-I (10 U/µl (Invitrogen; cat#18010-017)
- T4 DNA polymerase (5 U/µl Invitrogen; cat#18005-025)
- *E. coli* DNA ligase (10 U/µl Invitrogen cat#18052-019)
- 10x T7 RNA polymerase mix (comes with the Megascript kit)

Primers
- Oligo-dT-T7 primer (5'-AAA CGA CGG CCA GTG AAT TGT AAT ACG ACT CAC TAT AGG CGC T$_{(15)}$-3') (0.125-0.25 µg/µl for the first-round amplification depending on the amount of input total RNA and 0.5 µg/µl for the second-round amplification) in RNase free water. Synthesized primer should be SDS-PAGE purified to insure the full length. The concentration of primer is varied according to the starting material used. This promoter sequence is much longer than the consensus sequence defined by Dunn and Studier (1983) and can be purchased from New England Biolabs and Stratagene Inc. In the extended sequence shown here, the consensus sequence is embedded in the between a 5'flanking region that provides space for the T7 RNA polymerase to bind and a 3'-flanking trinucleotide that stimulates transcription catalyzed by the enzyme.
- TS primer (5' AAG CAG TGG TAA CAA CGC AGA GTA CGC GGG 3') (0.25 µg/µl) SDS-PAGE purified. According to the Chenchik's (ref. 73) data, ribounucleotide GGG at the 3' end should give the best TS effect instead of deoxinucleotide GGG. We have used TS primer with dGGG at the 3' end in multiple experiments and achieved satisfying results. The amount of TS primer used in the second-strand synthesis can be varied according to the amount of starting material. We generally use 0.25 µg/µl when 3-6 µg of total RNA used and 0.125 µg/µl when less total RNA used.
- Random hexamers (dN$_6$) (8 µg/µl).

Columns
- Micro Bio-Spin Chromatograph column (Bio-gel P-6) (Bio-Rad; Cat# 732-6222)
- Microcon YM-30 column (Millipore; Cat# 42410)

Procedures

First-Strand cDNA Synthesis

Template Switch Protocol
In PCR reaction tube, mix 0.01-5 µg total RNA in 8.5 µl DEPC H2O with 1 µl (0.1-0.25 µg/µl) oligo-dT(15)-T7 primer (5'-AAA CGA CGG CCA GTG AAT TGT AAT ACG ACT

CAC TAT AGG CGC T$_{(15)}$-3'), 1 µl of RNasin Plus and heat to 70°C for 3 min. Cool to room temperature then add the following reagents (a master mix can be prepared for multiple samples):
- 4 µl 5x first-strand buffer
- 1 µl (0.1-0.25 µg/µl) TS (template switch) oligo primer
- 2 µl 0.1 M DTT
- 2 µl 10 mM dNTP
- 1 µl Superscript-II
- 0.5 µl of T4gp32 (8 µg/µl)

Incubate at 50°C for 90 min in thermal cycler.

Eberwine's Protocol with Modification

In PCR reaction tube, mix 0.01-5 µg total RNA in 8.5 µl DEPC H2O with 1 µl (0.1-0.25 µg/µl) oligo-dT(24)-T7 primer (5'-AAA CGA CGG CCA GTG AAT TGT AAT ACG ACT CAC TAT AGG CGC T$_{(24)}$-3'), 1 µl of RNsin Plus and heat to 70°C for 3min. Cool to room temperature then add the following reagents (a master mix can be prepared for multiple samples):
- 4 µl 5x first-strand buffer
- 2 µl 0.1 M DTT
- 2 µl 10 mM dNTP
- 1 µl Superscript-II
- 0.5 µl of T4gp32 (8 µg/µl)

Incubate at 50°C for 90 min in thermal cycler.

Second-Strand cDNA Synthesis

Template Switch Protocol

Mix the following reagents:
- 106 µl of DEPC treated H$_2$O to the cDNA reaction tube
- 15 µl Advantage PCR buffer
- 3 µl 10 mM dNTP mix
- 1 µl of RNase-H
- 3 µl Advantage cDNA Polymerase mix

Cycle at 37°C for 5 min to digest mRNA, 94°C for 2 min to denature, 65°C for 1 min for specific priming and 75°C for 30 min for extension.[a]

Eberwine's Protocol with Modification

Mix the following reagents:
- 89 µl of DEPC treated H$_2$O to the cDNA reaction tube
- 30 µl 10x second-strand buffer
- 3 µl 10 mM dNTP mix
- 1 µl of RNase-H
- 4 µl of *E. coli* DNA polymerase-I (40U)
- 1 µl of *E. coli* DNA Ligase (10U)

Incubate at 15°C for 2 hours. Then, add 2 µl of T4 DNA polymerase (20U) and incubate at 15°C for 5 min.[b]

Stop the reaction with 7.5 µl 1 M NaOH solution containing 2 mM EDTA and incubate at 65°C for 10 min to inactivate enzymes. Reaction can be stopped after this step and the reaction tube can be stored at -20°C.

---

[a] Since the TS primer that initiates the second-strand cDNA synthesis is already present in the first-strand cDNA synthesis reaction and has been primed to the extended part of the cDNA, no additional primer is required in this step.

[b] From here on the steps are all the same for both template switch and Eberwine's protocols, unless specified.

Double Stranded cDNA Clean-Up

This step is designed to prevent carry over of nonincorporated dNTP, primers and inactivated enzymes into the following in vitro transcription. Keep in mind that although the double stranded cDNAs are stable and will not be affected by RNase contamination, they will be used as template in the IVT reaction, which should be RNase free.

Phenol-Chloroform-Isoamyl Isolation and Ethanol Precipitation

Add 1 µl linear Acrylamide (0.1 µg/µl) as DNA carrier to the sample to enhance double-stranded cDNA precipitation. Add 150 µl Phenol:Chloroform:Isoamyl alcohol (25:24:1) to the double stranded cDNA tube and mix well by pipetting (be careful not to spill or contaminate). Transfer the slurry solution to Phase lock gel tube and spin at 14,000 rpm for 5 min at room temperature. Transfer the aqueous phase to RNase/DNase-free 1.7 ml tube and add 70 µl of 7.5 M ammonium acetate first and then 1 ml 100% ethanol (EtOH). Mix well. Centrifuge right away at 14,000 rpm for 20 min at room temperature to prevent coprecipitation of oligos. A visible small white pellet should be seen at the bottom of the tube even if nano grams of starting material have been used. This pellet suggests successful precipitation. Wash pellet with 800 µl 100% EtOH and spin down at maximum speed for 8 min. Repeat this washing step one more time. Air dry or speedvacand resuspend double stranded cDNA in 8 ul DEPC H$_2$O.

In Vitro Transcription (Ambion; T7 Megascript Kit #1334)

Mix the following reagents:
- 2 µl of each 75 mM NTP (A, G, C and UTP)
- 2 µl reaction buffer
- 2 µl enzyme mix (RNase inhibitor and T7 phage RNA polymerase)
- 8 µl double stranded cDNA

Incubate at 37°C for 5 hours. Incubation can be interrupted by storing reaction tube at − 20°C and resuming the incubation later on without losing efficiency.

Purification of Amplified RNA

Any manufactured RNA isolation kit can be applied. Monophasic reagent such as TRIzol reagent from GibcoBRL, (cat#15596) are used here based on the efficient recovery of aRNA. RNeasy mini kit could be used for aRNA purification instead of TRIzol but, in our experience, RNA recovering is about 50% of that recovered with the TRIzol method. Take the following steps:
- Add 0.5 ml of TRIzol solution to the transcription reaction. Mix the reagents well by pipetting or gently vortexing
- Add 100 µl chloroform. Mix the reagents by inverting the tube for 15 sec. Allow the tube to stand at room temperature for 2-3 min
- Centrifuge the tube at 10,000 g for 15 min at 4°C
- Transfer the aqueous phase to a fresh tube and add 250 µl of isopropanol
- Store the sample on ice for 5 min and then centrifuge at 10,000 g for 15 min
- Wash the pellet twice with 800 µl 70% EtOH
- Allow the pellet to dry in air on ice and then dissolve it in 20 µl DEPC H$_2$O
- Measure the quantity of RNA concentration spectrophotometrically

Second Round of Amplification

Mix amplified aRNA (0.5-1 µg) in 8 µl DEPC H$_2$O with 1 µl (2 µg/µl) random hexamer (i.e., dN6) and heat to 70°C for 3 min, then cool to room temperature. Then add the following reagents:
- 4 µl 5x first-strand buffer
- 1 µl (0.5 µg/µl) oligo-dT-T7 primer
- 2 µl 0.1 M DTT

- 1 μl RNAsin
- 2 μl 10mM dNTP
- 1 μl Superscript-II

Incubate at 42°C for 90 min.[c,d]

From here, follow the second strand cDNA synthesis, ds-cDNA clean-up. 40 μl IVT reaction is suggested for the second IVT. RNA isolation use 1 ml TRIzol as manual instructed.

Target Labeling by Reverse Transcription

Mix the following reagents:

- 4 μl first-strand buffer
- 1 μl dN6 primer (8 μg/μl)
- 2 μl 10X low-T dNTP (5 mM A, C and GTP, 2 mM dTTP)
- 2 μl Cy-dUTP (1 mM Cy3 or Cy5)
- 2 μl 0.1 M DTT
- 1 μl RNasin
- 3-6 μg amplified aRNA in 7 μl DEPC H_2O

Mix well and heat to 65°C for 5 min then cool down to 42°C.

Add 1.5 μl SSII. Incubate for 90 min at 42°C. Add 2.5 μl 0.5 M EDTA and heat to 65°C for 1 min. Add 5 μl 1 M NaOH and incubate at 65°C for 15 min to hydrolyze RNA. Add 12.5 μl 1M Tris immediately to neutralize the pH. Bring volume to 70 μl by adding 35 μl of 1x TE.[e]

Target Clean-Up

Prepare Bio-6 column and run target solution through it. Collect flow through and add 250 μl 1x TE to it. Concentrate target to ~20 μl using Microcon YM-30 column.

Hybridization

Combine Cy3 labeled reference sample and Cy5 labeled target sample (adjust the color to purple) and then complete dry the sample using speedvac. Resuspend sample in 37 μl volume containing 1 μl 50x Denhardt's blocking solution, 1 μl poly-dA (8 μg/μl), 1 μl yeast tRNA (4 μg/μl), 10 μl Human Cot-I DNA, 3 μl 20x SSC, 1 μl of 10% SDS and 20 μl of DEPC treated water. Heat sample for 2 min at 99°C and apply target mixture to array slide, add coverslip, place in humidified hybridization chamber, and hybridize at 65°C over night.

Slide Washing

To wash slides, take the following steps:

- Wash with 2x SSC + 0.1% SDS to get rid of the cover slide
- Wash with 1x SSC for 1 min
- Wash with 0.2x SSC for 1 min
- Wash with 0.05x SSC for 10 sec
- Centrifuge slide(s) at 80-100 g for 3 min. Slides can be put in slide rack on microplate carriers or in 50 ml conical tube and centrifuged in swinging-bucket rotor.

Slides are now ready for scanning!

---

[c] From here, follow the previously described procedure for second-strand cDNA synthesis (TS protocol or Eberwine protocol), double stranded cDNA cleanup. In the second IVT, 40 ml of IVT reaction mixture are suggested to use instead of 20 ml. RNA isolation is followed.

[d] More than 1 μg of aRNA is not suggested. Too much template in IVT reaction could cause the amplification to reach a plateau with loss of amplification linearity.

[e] The amounts of aRNA used for labeling depends on the size of the array. If the array with 2,000-8,000 genes, 3 mg aRNA will be sufficient while a larger chip such as 16-20 K will need 6 mg of aRNA. The labeling reaction components do not need to be changed.

References

1. Bittner M, Meltzer P, Chen Y et al. Molecular classification of cutaneous malignant melanoma by gene expression: Shifting from a countinuous spectrum to distinct biologic entities. Nature 2000; 406:536-840.
2. Wang E, Panelli MC, Marincola FM. Genomic analysis of cancer. Princ Pract Oncol 2003; 17(9):1-16.
3. Yeoh E-J, Ross ME, Shurtleff SA et al. Classification, subtype discovery and prediction of outcome in pediatric acute lymphoblastic leukemia by gene expression profiling. Cancer Cell 2002; 1:133-136.
4. Wang E, Miller LD, Ohnmacht GA et al. Prospective molecular profiling of subcutaneous melanoma metastases suggests classifiers of immune responsiveness. Cancer Res 2002; 62:3581-3586.
5. Panelli MC, Wang E, Phan G et al. Genetic profiling of peripheral mononuclear cells and melanoma metastases in response to systemic interleukin-2 administration. Genome Biol 2002; 3(7):(Research0035).
6. Wang E, Lichtenfels R, Bukur J et al. Ontogeny and oncogenesis balance the transcriptional profile of renal cell cancer. Cancer Res 2004; 64(20):7279-7287.
7. Wang E, Ngalame Y, Panelli MC et al. Peritoneal and sub-peritoneal stroma may facilitate regional spread of ovarian cancer. Clin Cancer Res 2005; 11(1):113-122.
8. Singh D, Febbo PG, Ross K et al. Gene expression correlates of clinical prostate cancer behavior. Cancer Cell 2002; 1(2):203-209.
9. Mellick AS, Day CJ, Weinstein SR et al. Differential gene expression in breast cancer cell lines and stroma-tumor differences in microdissected breast cancer biopsies by display array analysis. Int J Cancer 2002; 100:172-180.
10. Islam TC, Lindvall J, Wennborg A et al. Expression profiling in transformed human B cells: Influence of Btk mutations and comparison to B cell lymphomas using filter and oligonucleotide arrays. Eur J Immunol 2002; 32(4):982-993.
11. Sasaki H, Ide N, Fukai I et al. Gene expression analysis of human thymoma correlates with tumor stage. Int J Cancer 2002; 101(4):342-347.
12. Skotheim RI, Monni O, Mousses S et al. New insights into testicular germ cell tumorigenesis from gene expression profiling. Cancer Res 2002; 62(8):2359-2364.
13. DeRisi J, Penland L, Brown PO et al. Use of cDNA microarray to analyse gene expression patterns in human cancer. Nat Genet 1996; 14:457-460.
14. Wang E, Marincola FM. A natural history of melanoma: Serial gene expression analysis. Immunol Today 2000; 21(12):619-623.
15. Wang E, Marincola FM. cDNA microarrays and the enigma of melanoma immune responsiveness. Cancer J Sci Am 2001; 7(1):16-23.
16. Bonner RF, Emmert-Buck M, Cole K et al. Laser capture microdissection: Molecular analysis of tissue. Science 1997; 278(5342):1481,1483.
17. Pappalardo PA, Bonner R, Krizman DB et al. Microdissection, microchip arrays, and molecular analysis of tumor cells (primary and metastases). Semin Radiat Oncol 1998; 8(3):217-223.
18. St Croix B, Rago C, Velculescu V et al. Genes expressed in human tumor endothelium. Science 2000; 289(5482):1121-1122.
19. Tsuda H, Birrer MJ, Ito YM et al. Identification of DNA copy number changes in microdissected serous ovarian cancer tissue using a cDNA microarray platform. Cancer Genet Cytogenet 2004; 155(2):97-107.
20. Chen JJ, Wu R, Yang PC et al. Profiling expression patterns and isolating differentially expressed genes by cDNA microarray system with colorimetry detection. Genomics 1998; 51(3):313-324.
21. Rajeevan MS, Dimulescu IM, Unger ER et al. Chemiluminescent analysis of gene expression on high-density filter arrays. J Histochem Cytochem 1999; 47(3):337-342.
22. Zejie Y, Xiaoyi W, Yu T et al. The method of micro-displacement measurement to improve the space resolution of array detector. Med Engineer Phys 1998; 20:149-151.
23. Yu J, Othman MI, Farjo R et al. Evaluation and optimization of procedures for target labeling and hybridization of cDNA microarrays. Mol Vis 2002; 8:130-137.
24. Lockhart DJ, Dong H, Byrne MC et al. Expression monitoring of hybridization to high-density oligonucleotide arrays. Nature Biotechnol 1996; 14:1675-1680.
25. Luo L, Salunga RC, Guo H et al. Gene expression profiles of laser-captured adjacent neuronal subtypes. Nat Med 1999; 5(1):117-122.
26. Trenkle T, Welsh J, Jung B et al. Nonstoichiometric reduced complexity probes for cDNA arrays. Nucleic Acids Res 1998; 26(17):3883-3891.
27. Roozemond RC. Ultramicrochemical determination of nucleic acids in individual cells using the Zeiss UMSP-I microspectrophotometer. Application to isolated rat hepatocytes of different ploidy classes. Histochem J 1976; 8(6):625-638.

28. Uemura E. Age-related changes in neuronal RNA content in rhesus monkeys (Macaca mulatta). Brain Res Bull 1980; 5(2):117-119.
29. Skrypina NA, Timofeeva AV, Khaspekov GL et al. Total RNA suitable for molecular biology analysis. J Biotechnol 2003; 105(1-2):1-9.
30. Eberwine JH, Yeh H, Miyashiro K et al. Analysis of gene expression in single live neurons. Proc Natl Acad Sci USA 1992; 89:3010-3014.
31. Phillips J, Eberwine JH. Antisense RNA amplification: A linear amplification method for analyzing the mRNA population from single living cells. Methods 1996; 10(3):283-288.
32. Eberwine JH. Amplification of mRNA populations using aRNA generated from immobilized oligo(dT)-T7 primed cDNA. Biotechniques 1996; 20(4):584-594.
33. Wang E, Miller L, Ohnmacht GA et al. High fidelity mRNA amplification for gene profiling using cDNA microarrays. Nature Biotech 2000; 17(4):457-459.
34. Wang E, Marincola FM. Amplification of small quantities of mRNA for transcript analysis. In: Bowtell D, Sambrook J, eds. DNA Arrays - A Molecular Cloning Manual. Cold Springs Harbor: Cold Spring Harbor Laboratory Press, 2002:204-213.
35. Spiess AN, Mueller N, Ivell R. Amplified RNA degradation in T7-amplification methods results in biased microarray hybridizations. BMC Genomics 2003; 4(1):44.
36. Xiang CC, Chen M, Ma L et al. A new strategy to amplify degraded RNA from small tissue samples for microarray studies. Nucleic Acids Res 2003; 31(9):e53.
37. Malboeuf CM, Isaacs SJ, Tran NH et al. Thermal effects on reverse transcription: Improvement of accuracy and processivity in cDNA synthesis. Biotechniques 2001; 30(5):1074-8, (1080, 1082, passim).
38. Kenzelmann M, Klaren R, Hergenhahn M et al. High-accuracy amplification of nanogram total RNA amounts for gene profiling. Genomics 2004; 83(4):550-558.
39. Schlingemann J, Thuerigen O, Ittrich C et al. Effective transcriptome amplification for expression profiling on sense-oriented oligonucleotide microarrays. Nucleic Acids Res 2005; 33(3):e29.
40. Mizuno Y, Carninci P, Okazaki Y et al. Increased specificity of reverse transcription priming by trehalose and oligo-blockers allows high-efficiency window separation of mRNA display. Nucleic Acids Res 1999; 27(5):1345-1349.
41. Spiess AN, Mueller N, Ivell R. Trehalose is a potent PCR enhancer: Lowering of DNA melting temperature and thermal stabilization of taq polymerase by the disaccharide trehalose. Clin Chem 2004; 50(7):1256-1259.
42. Carninci P, Nishiyama Y, Westover A et al. Thermostabilization and thermoactivation of thermolabile enzymes by trehalose and its application for the synthesis of full length cDNA. Proc Natl Acad Sci USA 1998; 95(2):520-524.
43. Rapley R. Enhancing PCR amplification and sequencing using DNA-binding proteins. Mol Biotechnol 1994; 2(3):295-298.
44. Villalva C, Touriol C, Seurat P et al. Increased yield of PCR products by addition of T4 gene 32 protein to the SMART PCR cDNA synthesis system. Biotechniques 2001; 31(1):81-3, (86).
45. Van Gelder RN, von Zastrow ME, Yool A et al. Amplified RNA synthesized from limited quantities of heterogeneous cDNA. Proc Natl Acad Sci USA 1990; 87:1663-1667.
46. Baugh LR, Hill AA, Brown EL et al. Quantitative analysis of mRNA amplification by in vitro transcription. Nucleic Acids Res 2000; 29(5):E29-E38.
47. Gubler U, Hoffman BJ. A simple and very efficient method for generating cDNA libraries. Gene 1983; 25:263-269.
48. Li Y, Li T, Liu S et al. Systematic comparison of the fidelity of aRNA, mRNA and T-RNA on gene expression profiling using cDNA microarray. J Biotechnol 2004; 107(1):19-28.
49. Rudnicki M, Eder S, Schratzberger G et al. Reliability of t7-based mRNA linear amplification validated by gene expression analysis of human kidney cells using cDNA microarrays. Nephron Exp Nephrol 2004; 97(3):e86-e95.
50. Park JY, Kim SY, Lee JH et al. Application of amplified RNA and evaluation of cRNA targets for spotted-oligonucleotide microarray. Biochem Biophys Res Commun 2004; 325(4):1346-1352.
51. Li Y, Ali S, Philip PA et al. Direct comparison of microarray gene expression profiles between nonamplification and a modified cDNA amplification procedure applicable for needle biopsy tissues. Cancer Detect Prev 2003; 27(5):405-411.
52. Kacharmina JE, Crino PB, Eberwine JH. Preparation of cDNA from single cells and subcellular regions. Methods Enzymol 1999; 303:3-19.
53. Matz M, Shagin D, Bogdanova E et al. Amplification of cDNA ends based on template-switching effect and step-out PCR. Nucleic Acids Res 1999; 27(6):1558-1560.
54. Chenchik A, Zhu YY, Diatchenko L et al. Generation and use of high-quality cDNA from small amounts of total RNA by SMART(TM) PCR. In: Siebert P, Larrick J, eds. Gene Cloning and Analysis by RT-PCR. Natick: Biotechniques Books, 1998:305-319.

55. Zhao H, Hastie T, Whitfield ML et al. Optimization and evaluation of T7 based RNA linear amplification protocols for cDNA microarray analysis. BMC Genomics 2002; 3(1):31.
56. Marko NF, Frank B, Quackenbush J et al. A robust method for the amplification of RNA in the sense orientation. BMC Genomics 2005; 6(1):27.
57. Goff LA, Bowers J, Schwalm J et al. Evaluation of sense-strand mRNA amplification by comparative quantitative PCR. BMC Genomics 2004; 5(1):76.
58. Cheetham GM, Jeruzalmi D, Steitz TA. Transcription regulation, initiation, and "DNA scrunching" by T7 RNA polymerase. Cold Spring Harb Symp Quant Biol 1998; 63:263-267.
59. Feldman AL, Costouros NG, Wang E et al. Advantages of mRNA amplification for microarray analysis. Biotechniques 2002; 33(4):906-914.
60. Gold D, Coombes K, Medhane D et al. A comparative analysis of data generated using two different target preparation methods for hybridization to high-density oligonucleotide microarrays. BMC Genomics 2004; 5(1):2.
61. Polz MF, Cavanaugh CM. Bias in template-to-product ratios in multitemplate PCR. Appl Environ Microbiol 1998; 64(10):3724-3730.
62. Seth D, Gorrell MD, McGuinness PH et al. SMART amplification maintains representation of relative gene expression: Quantitative validation by real time PCR and application to studies of alcoholic liver disease in primates. J Biochem Biophys Methods 2003; 55(1):53-66.
63. Smith L, Underhill P, Pritchard C et al. Single primer amplification (SPA) of cDNA for microarray expression analysis. Nucleic Acids Res 2003; 31(3):e9.
64. Bettinotti MP, Panelli MC, Ruppe E et al. Clinical and immunological eveluation of patients with metastatic melanoma undergoing immunization with the HLA-C2*0702 associated epitope MAGE-A12:170-178. Int J Cancer 2003; 105:210-216.
65. Iscove NN, Barbara M, Gu M et al. Representation is faithfully preserved in global cDNA amplified exponentially from sub-picogram quantities of mRNA. Nature Biotech 2002; 20:940-943.
66. Stirewalt DL, Pogosova-Agadjanyan EL, Khalid N et al. Single-stranded linear amplification protocol results in reproducible and reliable microarray data from nanogram amounts of starting RNA. Genomics 2004; 83(2):321-331.
67. Petalidis L, Bhattacharyya S, Morris GA et al. Global amplification of mRNA by template-switching PCR: Linearity and application to microarray analysis. Nucleic Acids Res 2003; 31(22):e142.
68. Rox JM, Bugert P, Muller J et al. Gene expression analysis in platelets from a single donor: Evaluation of a PCR-based amplification technique. Clin Chem 2004; 50(12):2271-2278.
69. Klur S, Toy K, Williams MP et al. Evaluation of procedures for amplification of small-size samples for hybridization on microarrays. Genomics 2004; 83(3):508-517.
70. Ohtsuka S, Iwase K, Kato M et al. An mRNA amplification procedure with directional cDNA cloning and strand-specific cRNA synthesis for comprehensive gene expression analysis. Genomics 2004; 84(4):715-729.
71. Randolph JB, Waggoner AS. Stability, specificity and fluorescence brightness of multiply-labeled fluorescent DNA probes. Nucleic Acids Res 1997; 25(14):2923-2929.
72. DeRisi J. Stability, specificity and fluorescence brightness of mulitply-labeled fluorescent DNA probes. In: Bowtell D, Sambrook J, eds. DNA Arrays - A Molecular Cloning Manual. Cold Spring Harbor: Cold Spring Harbor Laboratory Press, 2002:204-213.
73. Chenchik A, Zhu YY, Diatchenko L et al. Generation and use of high-quality cDNA from small amounts of total RNA bby SMARTTM PCR. In: Siebert P, Larrick J, eds. Gene cloning and analysis by RT-PCR. Eaton Publishing Company/Biotechniques, 1998:305-319.

Complementary Techniques:
Laser Capture Microdissection—Increasing Specificity of Gene Expression Profiling of Cancer Specimens

Giovanni Esposito*

Abstract

Recent developments in sensitive genome characterization and quantitative gene expression analyses that permit precise molecular genetic fingerprinting of tumoral tissue are having a huge impact on cancer diagnostics. However, the significance of the data obtained with these techniques strictly depends on the composition of the biological sample to be analyzed and is greatly enhanced by including a preprocessing step that allows the researcher to distinguish and isolate selected cell populations from surrounding undesired material. This may represent a remarkable problem: indeed, genomic and proteomic analysis in the context of cancer investigation is susceptible to contamination by nonneoplastic cells, which can mask some tumor-specific alterations. Moreover, the heterogeneity of the tissues of a histological section, in which the cell population of interest may constitute only a small fraction, can represent an insurmountable difficulty for the use of quantitative techniques that absolutely depend on genomic material strictly derived from the cells that require analysis. This is obviously not possible if DNA or RNA is extracted from entire biopsies.

In the past, this obstacle was partially overcome by manual dissection from slides with a needle or scalpel; however, this method is feasible only if there is a clear demarcation between the tissue under consideration and its surroundings and moreover, allows only an approximate separation of tissues. The recent development of microdissection systems based on laser technology has largely solved this important problem.

Laser microdissection is a powerful tool for the isolation of specific cell populations (or single cells) from stained sections of both formalin-fixed, paraffin-embedded and frozen tissues, from cell cultures and even of a single chromosome within a metaphase cell. Resulting material is suitable for a wide range of downstream assays such LOH (loss of heterozygosity) studies, gene expression analysis at the mRNA level and a variety of proteomic approaches such as 2D gel analysis, reverse phase protein array and SELDI protein profiling. This chapter describes the characteristics of the most widely utilized laser microdissection systems and their current applications.

Microdissection Technologies: The Past and the Present

The shift from the concept of cellular pathology, formulated by the German pathologist Rudolf Virchow in the second half of the 19th century, to the current concept of molecular pathology, made possible by remarkable developments in the knowledge of the molecular

*Giovanni Esposito—Department of Oncological and Surgical Sciences, University of Padova, via Gattamelata 64, 35128 Padova, Italy. Email: giovanni.esposito@unipd.it

Microarray Technology and Cancer Gene Profiling, edited by Simone Mocellin.
©2007 Landes Bioscience and Springer Science+Business Media.

processes involved in human disease achieved in recent years through molecular biology techniques, represents the latest of several revolutions that pathological anatomy has faced during its long history. It appears now clear that, in the future, the skills of the pathologist and those of the molecular biologist will have to be more integrated. Laser microdissection is, without doubt, a key technique in this perspective.

The need to isolate specific cellular types from complex tissues with the aim of carrying out accurate molecular assays has been argued for decades. Beginning in the 1970s, several papers have described different techniques to accomplish this task. They were based on the manual dissection (under microscope control) using razor blades, needles or fine glass pipettes to isolate the cells of interest from the rest of the section.[1-4] However, manual dissection is too time consuming and moreover, it does not allow precise control of the material effectively selected. In the last decade, attempts have therefore been made to standardize more efficient techniques. A significant technological advance in microdissection procedures was proposed in 1993 by Shibata.[5] He published a study which described a technique that relied on a negative selection of material (SURF: Selective Ultraviolet Radiation Fractionation): this technique used an UV laser beam in order to destroy the DNA of all the undesired components of the tissue, while the cells to be studied were protected from the action of the laser by a dye. Obviously, this technique was applicable only for molecular analysis of DNA.

Subsequent improvements led to the development of more sophisticated techniques, all based on a laser beam and able to isolate even one single cell, with the possibility to obtain DNA, RNA or proteins for molecular studies.

In 1996, Emmert-Buck and colleagues of the National Institutes of Health (NIH) in Bethesda, MD, introduced the LCM (Laser Capture Microdissection) system,[6] which was later commercialized by Arcturus Engineering as the PixCell System. Other companies subsequently developed new systems for laser microdissection, with various characteristics regarding the method to collect cells, the laser, etc. Today, the systems produced by Arcturus Engineering, P.A.L.M. Microlaser Technologies and Leica Microsystems are among the most popular. The following section outlines the functional characteristics of these three systems, with the reminder that they are continuously being updated (Fig. 1).

Arcturus System (PixCell)

The LCM system by Arcturus utilizes a low-power infrared laser to melt a special thermoplastic film (ethylene vinyl acetate membrane - EVA) on top of the cells to be isolated. A glass slide with the sectioned tissue is placed on the stage of the microscope and an area of interest is selected by the user on a computer screen. A custom-designed PCR- tube cap, coated with thermoplastic film, is then placed on the tissue section by means of a transport arm. The laser is then directed through the cap to melt the film onto the target cells. Pulsing the laser through the cap causes the thermoplastic film to form a thin protrusion that bridges the gap between the cap and the tissue and adheres to the targeted cells: in this way they are embedded by the polymer. The laser diameter can be adjusted from 7.5 to 30 μm so that individual cells, or an entire cluster of cells, can be selected. When the cap is lifted off the tissue section, the selected cells are attached and captured, ready to be transferred into a microfuge tube containing the appropriate extraction buffer for further analyses. The rest of the section remains intact and ready for further dissections. The morphology of the transferred cells is preserved and can be visualized under the microscope. The entire process is easily documented by means of a database program able to record images of both the area of interest and the dissected cells. This system has the unquestionable advantage of being able to use normal glass slides and therefore, theoretically, material prepared routinely for diagnostic purposes is also utilizable, obviously after removing the coverslip. A problem in common with all microdissection methods is its suboptimal microscopic visualisation because of the absence of a mounting medium and a coverslip. However, this shortcoming does not pose a problem when the identification of the cell types for microdissection is performed by an experienced pathologist.

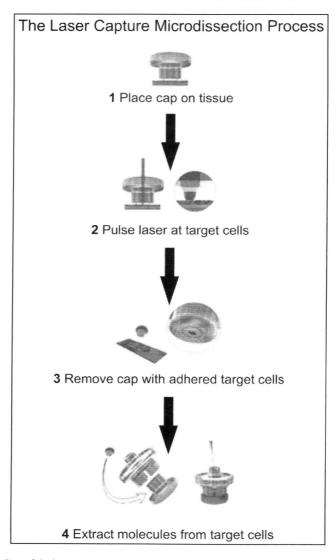

Figure 1A. Outline of the laser microdissection systems' characteristics: 1A) Arcturus Pixcell.

Arcturus has recently commercialized a new system (Veritas™ microdissection) that combines the LCM system, based on infrared laser, with UV laser cutting.

(For more details, go to the following web site: www.arctur.com.)

P.A.L.M. System (MicroBeam)

The system of P.A.L.M. Microlaser Technologies is based on the Laser Microdissection and Pressure Catapulting (LMPC) technology. Mounted on an inverted microscope, the system selects the areas of interest in tissue sections mounted on a microscope slide coated by a Polyethylennaphtalate (PEN) membrane and catapults them into a collection tube by means of a pulsed ultra-violet (UV-A, 337 nm wavelength) laser. This laser is coupled with the

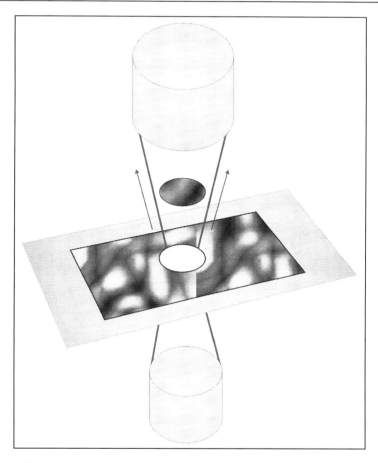

Figure 1B.Outline of the laser microdissection systems' characteristics: P.A.L.M. Laser microdissection and pressure catapulting (LMPC).

inverted microscope and focused through the objective lenses to a micron-sized spot diameter. The narrow laser focal spot allows the ablation of the material while the surrounding tissue remains fully intact. At the focal point, unwanted material is photo fragmented into molecules and atoms, a phenomenon called "cold ablation".[7] Photo ablation was first described by Srinivasan, who used the ablative forces of an excimer laser to ablate polymers.[8] He later employed the ablative photodecomposition device (APD) for the ablation of biological matter.[9] The focused laser leaves nothing behind that could be analyzed as a bio molecule. All the matter onto which the laser is focused is in the state of fragments of molecules, ions or other debris, cut into remnants of low molecular weight or even atoms. Since this cutting is a fast, photochemical process without heat transfer, the adjacent biological matter or bio molecules such as DNA, RNA and proteins are not affected. Moreover, the 337 nm nitrogen laser works within an UV-A range, where no damage of biological matter occurs. Therefore, these molecules can be isolated from the specimen for downstream analyses and applications. The noncontact capture of homogeneous tissue samples or individual cells is achieved by means of catapulting using P.A.L.M.'s patented Laser Pressure Catapulting technology. With the same laser, the separated cells, or the selected tissue area, can be directly catapulted into the cap of a common microfuge tube in an entirely noncontact procedure with the help of a single

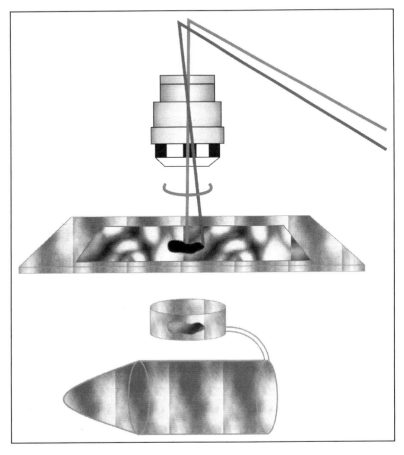

Figure 1C.Outline of the laser microdissection systems' characteristics: Leica AS LMD (modified from respective web sites).

defocused laser pulse. The sample is driven at high speed along the wave front of the powerful photonic stream and can be "beamed" several millimetres away, even against gravity.

(For more details, go to the following web site: www.palm-microlaser.com).

Leica System (AS LMD)

The Leica AS LMD Laser Microdissection System is based on an automated laboratory microscope integrated with an UV laser. Through this system, the tissue sections that are to be microdissected are mounted on polyethylennaphtalate (PEN)-foiled slides, which are microscope glass slides that support a thin plastic (PEN) film (cell culture samples are grown in special Petri dishes with a PEN surface). After selecting the area of interest on a computer screen, a pulsed UV-A laser (337.1 nm wavelength) cuts the plastic film by "cold ablation" along the drawn line and the excised section falls by gravity into a PCR-tube cap located directly beneath the slide. This technique avoids direct UV irradiation of the dissected cells (even if no interaction with DNA or RNA and UV radiation used would take place) or mechanical contact that could cause contamination. The result of the cutting can be easily checked by an automated inspection mode. To perform the cut, the laser beam moves over the specimen, with its direction along the cutting line controlled by two rotating prisms. In this

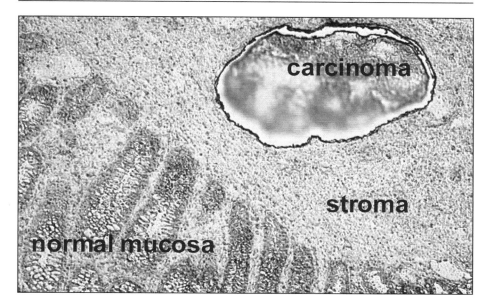

Figure 2A. Selective microdissection of neoplastic cells from a frozen section of primary colon cancer stained with haematoxylin (Leica AS LMD - original magnification 10X): the laser cuts along the line drawn by the operator, isolating the neoplastic cells.

way, the specimen remains stable so that it can be clearly observed during the cutting process. All steps are documented by means of an image archiving software. (For more details, go to the following web site: www.leica-microsystems.com).

All three systems are equally able to isolate living cells, can be used in fluorescence and allow creation of a database of archived images.

Why Microdissection?

The aim of tissue microdissection is to select and isolate single cells or groups of cells from a heterogeneous tissue sample in order to perform molecular analyses. The development of tissue microdissection techniques and the increasing interest towards them are a consequence of the refinement of PCR techniques which permit molecular analyses from very limited amounts of biological material, but require very pure preparations to avoid any risk of contamination. Microdissection techniques are useful in the analysis of heterogeneous tissues containing numerous cell types. For instance, a tumor sample is obviously constituted of tumor cells, but also of stromal cells (fibroblasts and endothelial cells), inflammatory cells and red blood cells; some tumors, e.g., pancreatic adenocarcinoma, in which a prominent desmoplastic reaction and often an evident lymphocytic infiltrate are observable, the number of tumor cells may actually be much lower than that of the noncancerous cells. Conventional techniques for molecular analyses based on whole tissue dissociation therefore introduce an initial contamination problem that reduces the specificity and sensitivity of the downstream molecular techniques, thus making the interpretation of the results more difficult. On the contrary, laser microdissection represents an ideal method for the extraction of cells from samples in which the exact morphology of both isolated cells and surrounding tissues is observable and preserved (Fig. 2). In this way, laser microdissection represents a very interesting technique in molecular pathology and creates a link between histology and molecular analysis.

Due to limits connected to sample preservation methods described below, tissue microdissection is currently more widely employed to analyze DNA than RNA or proteins, which are

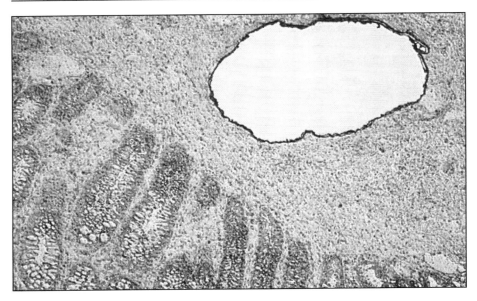

Figure 2B. Selective microdissection of neoplastic cells from a frozen section of primary colon cancer stained with haematoxylin (Leica AS LMD - original magnification 10X): the neoplastic cells fall into a PCR tube cap.

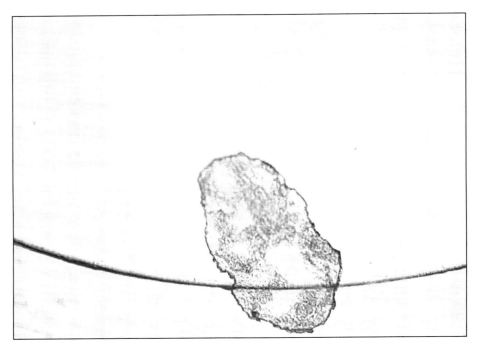

Figure 2C. Selective microdissection of neoplastic cells from a frozen section of primary colon cancer stained with haematoxylin (Leica AS LMD - original magnification 10X): inspection of the tube cap showing the isolated cells.

much more sensitive to degradation and fixation. However, tissue microdissected from carefully preserved frozen samples is suitable for protein analysis, and can also be employed for refined investigations of RNA expression using sensitive methods such as quantitative RT-PCR and microarray analysis.[10-18]

Microdissection is currently most commonly applied to analyze molecular alterations in tumors, with the majority of studies focused at the DNA level to detect loss of heterozygosity, microsatellite instability and the presence of mutations in tumor suppressor genes and oncogenes. In addition to enriching for tumor cells by eliminating surrounding stroma, microdissection permits comparison of distinct zones of tumor cells within a given lesion, the tumor cell population with neighboring normal cells and different stages of tumor progression coexisting in the same primary tumor sample (dysplasia, in situ carcinoma, invasive carcinoma) as well as metastases.

Laser microdissection can be applied to routinely formalin fixed - paraffin embedded tissues, frozen tissues, cytological preparations as well as cultured cells. Obviously, each one of these biological materials presents its own peculiarities and specific problems when dealing with the optimization of protocols upstream and downstream of microdissection.

In the case of histological preparations, it is certainly better to utilize samples that have been snap-frozen and stored in liquid nitrogen (or alternatively at -80°C). Formalin (4% buffered formaldehyde), the standard fixative routinely used in pathology laboratories, is an "additive" fixative that creates cross-links between itself and proteins and between nucleic acids and proteins. This can interfere with the recovery of nucleic acids and proteins, as well as with the amplification of DNA and RNA by PCR. As a consequence of these cross-links, the nucleic acids isolated from these specimens are highly fragmented, the extent of fragmentation mainly depending on the fixation conditions. This problem often occurs when using years-old archived material, especially since pathology laboratories did not pay much attention to fixation times in the past. In fact, the longer the fixation time, the stronger the cross-linking will become. The optimal fixation time in buffered formaldehyde solution is 24 hours. While fixation for up to 48 hours is still compatible with subsequent molecular analysis, soaking in formalin for more than 1 week destroys nucleic acids.

It is advisable to choose alcoholic rather than additive fixatives, as alcohols fix the tissues by dehydrating them but without creating chemical links; however, in the majority of laboratories, this is feasible only if microdissection is considered from the start as one of the possible options for processing the sample. Frozen sections obtained by cryostat cutting have the advantage of not undergoing cross-links due to fixatives but, on the other hand, show poor histological definition; not to mention that frozen material is not always easily obtainable.

For these reasons, it would be very important to find a standardized procedure that allows adequate extraction and eventual amplification of nucleic acids from routinely processed material. Some publications propose methods for this purpose. All these papers mainly deal with the problem of DNA fragmentation due to formalin fixation and the necessity for increased purity of the isolated nucleic acids. For instance, in a study of urinary bladder cancers and gliomas, Zhi-Ping Ren and coauthors[19] suggest that the key to successful DNA recovery is to completely digest all the proteins in the tissue sample. In their opinion, any leftover proteins associated with chromosomes would seriously affect the quality as well as the quantity of the DNA template. They underline the importance of strictly controlling the Proteinase K concentration and incubation time. The other side of this problem is the optimization of the PCR conditions. When dealing with formalin-fixed microdissected material, it is sometimes difficult to amplify the gene of interest using primer pairs that work very well for cell lines or fresh frozen materials. This is probably due to the fact that the DNA double helix has been broken into smaller fragments. This can be circumvented by employing a new set of primer pairs that amplifies a shorter fragment e.g., about 120 base pairs.

With these adjustments, the authors maintain that they were able to recover amplifiable DNA from virtually all investigated formalin-fixed, paraffin-embedded microdissected samples (99%).

The scenario regarding RNA extraction is quite different, as protocols that allow the use of RNA isolated from microdissected formalin-fixed paraffin-embedded cells require further improvements and validation.

The literature includes a few articles that describe RNA extraction from whole, fixed biopsies. Gloghini et al[20] published an interesting study that investigated whether RNA can be efficiently isolated from Bouin-fixed (a fixative that incorporates picric acid) or formalin-fixed lymphoid tissue specimens. Using a combination of Proteinase K digestion and column purification, they were able to obtain RNA that yielded accurate real time quantitative RT-PCR results.

Finally, it is important to remember that several companies have produced kits specifically devoted to the extraction of RNA from small amounts of material obtained by microdissection.

A product named RNAlater (Ambion - web site: www.ambion.com) is currently in wide use to improve RNA preservation in biological samples. RNAlater is an aqueous, nontoxic, tissue storage reagent that quickly permeates the tissues in order to stabilize and protect RNA in fresh specimens. RNAlater eliminates the need to immediately process or freeze the samples; the specimen can simply be submerged in RNAlater and stored for extended periods (up to 1 week at room temperature, 1 month at +4°C, indefinitely at -20°C) and thus allows the investigator to analyze the sample at a later time. While there is no doubt about the effectiveness of RNAlater in preserving nucleic acids from degradation, there are contrasting data about the product's effects on morphological preservation and subsequent microscopic observation.[21,22] In our experience, it is very difficult, if not impossible, to obtain satisfactory cryostat sections from some tissues, thus making RNAlater unsuitable for the preservation of samples destined to microdissection. Therefore, one needs to carefully choose the storage modality of the samples in connection with the type of analysis to be performed. As we have seen above, histological samples are routinely formalin fixed in clinical practice for diagnostic purposes. This procedure does not preserve DNA or RNA from degradation and cannot be used for proteomic analyses, since formalin extensively crosslinks proteins, thus preventing subsequent molecular studies.[23] Today pathologists understand the need to provide fresh tissue samples for research purposes, but the preservation method becomes of utmost importance in order to guarantee the feasibility of future molecular studies. The optimization of specific preservation methods compatible with the widest possible spectrum of assays on a given sample would be accelerated by the combined input of surgeons, pathologists and molecular biologists.

Slide Preparation for Microdissection

It is not the purpose of this chapter to provide a detailed description of technical procedures; the following are only indications about specific issues in slide preparation for laser microdissection.

The brochures provided by Arcturus, P.A.L.M. and Leica emphasise the possibility of utilizing routine standardized staining procedures, but recommend protocols characterised by very brief treatment times. In fact, in agreement with the rather obvious general rule that we have drawn—i.e., the least manipulation in the shortest time yields the best results—some adjustments are required in order to shorten the staining procedure, both for frozen and for fixed and embedded tissues.

If the material to be microdissected is destined for RNA extraction, care must be taken in order to create a ribonuclease (RNase)-free environment to avoid RNA degradation; RNases are ubiquitous, very stable and difficult to inactivate. Hand contact, laboratory glassware and dust particles are the most common sources of RNase contamination. To prevent contamination from these sources, it is necessary to wear powder-free gloves at all times when handling reagents and RNA samples and to sterilize glassware by heat. When dealing with frozen tissue, one must keep in mind that endogenous RNases may still be active even after short-time fixation phases. Therefore, it is advisable to keep all histochemistry incubation steps as short as possible. RNase-free water, solutions and ethanol series should be used. RNase-free solutions can be obtained by treatment with DEPC (diethylpyrocarbonate), which destroys the activity of RNases.

Another open issue regards the choice of the histological staining protocol. Ideally, staining should provide an acceptable morphology to allow the selection of target cells and without interfering with the macromolecules of interest or with the subsequent molecular techniques. A series of nuclear dyes have been examined but, up to now, they have not yielded univocal results. Ehrig et al[24] examined the effect of four dyes (methyl green, haematoxylin, toluidine blue O, azure B) on DNA extraction from fixed and frozen tissues. They concluded that DNA recovery from a microdissected tissue is not connected to the histological stain chosen. Burgemeister et al[25] compared haematoxylin/eosin, methylene blue, methyl green and nuclear fast red on frozen sections for RNA isolation. In their experience, the best results were achieved using methyl green and nuclear fast red stains; haematoxylin/eosin results were similar to nuclear fast red and methylene blue staining yielded partially degraded RNA. Okuducu et al[26] stained frozen sections from prostatic tissue with haematoxylin, methyl green, toluidine blue O and May-Grunwald in order to identify a reliable stain for RNA analysis. Results of real-time quantitative RT-PCR performed after laser microdissection showed that methyl green yielded more RT-PCR product than the other dyes. On the other hand, the main protocol provided by Leica suggests the use of haematoxylin but in an alternative protocol reports that there are indications of better PCR results when using methyl green or toluidine blue. Arcturus proposes its own kit, but does not specify the dye used. P.A.L.M. hosts customers' protocols on its website; for histological staining of frozen sections, a rapid haematoxylin stain is recommended.

Finally, haematoxylin and methyl green seem to have no effect on protein migration and therefore should be suitable for staining tissues to be microdissected for protein analyses.[27]

Sections prepared for microdissection are dehydrated and kept without a coverslip, which results in reduced cellular detail. This makes it hard to distinguish and isolate specific cell populations from lesions where morphologically similar cell types are strictly intermingled, such as lymphomas or carcinomas with a diffused growth pattern. Immunohistochemical staining of sections could help in identifying and isolating specific cell populations, even of identical morphology, according to their antigen expression, thus allowing a more precise microdissection. However, standard immunohistochemical staining protocols need several hours, which can lead to significant degradation of the macromolecules of interest, especially RNA by RNases activated in aqueous environments. In 1999, Fend et al[28,29] proposed a rapid immuno-staining procedure (total processing time from 12 to 25 minutes) for frozen sections followed by laser capture microdissection (LCM) and RNA extraction, which allows a targeted mRNA analysis of immunophenotypically defined cell populations. In 2000, Fink et al proposed the use of immunofluorescence applied to microdissection;[30,31] along this line of thought, a paper published by Burbach et al in 2004[32] described a rapid immunofluorescence staining approach combined with laser microdissection on frozen sections of mouse brain that does not interfere with RNA recovery and integrity for quantitative RT-PCR.

Another important issue concerns the number of cells that must be dissected. In the literature, this number ranges broadly, depending on the macromolecules to be analyzed, the methodology of their extraction (using "home-brewed" protocols or one of numerous commercial kits dedicated to extraction from small quantities of cells), the downstream bio molecular techniques adopted, fixed or frozen samples and last but not least, the operator's technical skill. When dealing with methods of linear RNA amplification, it is possible to perform gene expression profiling analyses even from a very limited number of cells, as the most critical parameters for the success of such an experiment seem to be the integrity and purity of the RNA.

In Our Laboratory

Our laboratory has direct experience with the Leica microdissection system, which is available in our Department. We have carried out a series of trials aimed at identifying the best conditions both for the conservation of the samples and to obtain an acceptable amount and quality of the extracted genomic material (DNA or RNA), which led us to introduce some modifications into the manufacturer's protocols. The following points concern the protocols that we now utilize in our laboratory.

Microdissection for DNA Extraction

DNA can be extracted from both frozen and formalin-fixed paraffin-embedded tissues. In the latter case, 4 μm microtome sections are obtained and mounted on polyethylennaphtalate (PEN)-foiled slides (Leica Microsystems). Immediately after slicing, the sections are placed at 60°C for 30 min, then de-paraffinazed in 3 histoclear baths (3 × 1 min), rehydrated in decreasing alcohols (100%, 95%, 70%, 50%, each for 30 seconds) and washed for 30 seconds in distilled water. They are then lightly stained with Mayer's haematoxylin (30 seconds), rapidly washed in tap water, stained with eosin for 30 seconds, rapidly washed in distilled water, dehydrated in increasing alcohols (70%, 95%, 100%, each for 30 seconds) and finally air dried for 10 minutes and microdissected at once.

Microdissection for RNA Extraction

In a cryostat set, snap-frozen specimens are anchored on cryostat supports using diethylpyrocarbonate (DEPC)-water (without OCT embedding) and sliced into 7-μm sections using a disposable blade. Immediately after slicing, the sections are fixed for 1 min in 70% alcohol, lightly stained with Mayer's haematoxylin (30 sec), washed in 2 DEPC-water baths (5 min each), dehydrated in increasing alcohols (80%, 95%, 100%), placed at 37°C for 30 min and then promptly microdissected. To suppress RNase activity, DEPC-water is also used for alcohol dilutions.

Another technical aspect concerns the possibility of storing slides at -20°C, or better at -80°C after the cryostat cut. This would allow the operator to perform the time-consuming microdissection at a later time or in more than one sitting, which would be especially helpful when a large number of small groups of cells need to be microdissected. To test this possibility, we prepared multiple sections from the same specimen and then stained and microdissected them either on the same day or after one day's storage at -80°C. Unfortunately, we found that the stored samples yielded much lower quantities of RNA compared to the freshly processed samples. Therefore, in our opinion, it is currently advisable to carry out all the phases of the microdissection process in the same day.

Conclusions

Laser microdissection is an extremely valuable tool for isolating and analyzing specific cell populations or subcellular material from sections of frozen tissues, paraffin embedded material, cytological preparations, living cells and even chromosome spreads. Coupled with state-of-the-art molecular analyses, the technique has already made a major contribution to studies aimed at understanding normal cell functions and at revealing the molecular changes underlying neo-plastic progression. With anticipated improvements in preservation and staining protocols, laser microdissection should become even more valuable in the future.

References

1. Abeln EC, Smit VT, Wessels JW et al. Molecular genetic evidence for the conversion hypothesis of the origin of malignant mixed mullerian tumours. J Pathol 1997; 183:424-31.
2. Perren A, Roth J, Muletta-Feurer S et al. Clonal analysis of sporadic pancreatic endocrine tumours. J Pathol 1998; 186:363-71.
3. Saxena A, Alport EC, Custead S et al. Molecular analysis of clonality of sporadic angiomyolipoma. J Pathol 1999; 189:79-84.
4. Looijenga LH, Rosemberg C, van Gurp RH et al. Comparative genomic hybridization of microdissected samples from different stages in the development of a seminoma and a non-seminoma. J Pathol 2000; 191:187-92.
5. Shibata D. Selective ultraviolet radiation fractionation and polymerase chain reaction analysis of genetic alterations. Am J Pathol 1993; 143:1523-6.
6. Emmert-Buck MR, Bonner RF, Smith PD et al. Laser capture microdissection. Science 1996; 274:998-1001.
7. Vogel A, Venugopalan V. Mechanisms of pulsed laser ablation of biological tissues. Chem Rev 2003; 103:577-644.

8. Srinivasan R, Leigh WJ. Ablative photodecomposition: Action of far ultraviolet (193 nm) laser radiation on poly (ethyleneterephthalate) films. J Amer Chem Soc 1982; 104:6784-5.
9. Trokel SL, Srinivasan R, Braren B. Excimer laser surgery of the cornea. Am J Ophthalmol 1983; 96:710-5.
10. Di Cristofano C, Mrad K, Zavaglia K et al. Papillary lesions of the breast: A molecular progression? Breast Cancer Res Treat 2005; 90:71-6.
11. D'Arrigo A, Belluco C, Ambrosi A et al. Metastatic transcriptional pattern revealed by gene expression profiling in primary colorectal carcinoma. Int J Cancer 2005; 115:256-62.
12. Coco S, Defferrari R, Scaruffi P et al. Genome analysis and gene expression profiling of neuroblastoma and ganglioneuroblastoma reveal differences between neuroblastic and Schwannian stromal cells. J Pathol 2005; 207:346-357.
13. Burgemeister R. New aspects of laser microdissection in research and routine. J Histochem Cytochem 2005; 53:409-12.
14. Schneider-Stock R, Boltze C, Jaeger V et al. Significance of loss of heterozygosity of the RB1 gene during tumour progression in well-differentiated liposarcomas. J Pathol 2002; 197:654-60.
15. Sethi N, Palefsky J. Transcriptional profiling of dysplastic lesions in K14-HPV16 transgenic mice using laser microdissection. FASEB J 2004; 18:1243-5.
16. Cowherd SM, Espina VA, Petricoin IIIrd EF et al. Proteomic analysis of human breast cancer tissue with laser-capture microdissection and reverse-phase protein microarrays. Clin Breast Cancer 2004; 5:385-92.
17. Sugiyama Y, Farrow B, Murillo C et al. Analysis of differential gene expression patterns in colon cancer and cancer stroma using microdissected tissues. Gastroenterology 2005; 128:480-6.
18. Ma XJ, Salunga R, Tuggle JT et al. Gene expression profiles of human breast cancer progression. Proc Natl Acad Sci USA 2003; 100:5974-9.
19. Ren ZP, Sallstrom J, Sundstrom C et al. Recovering DNA and optimizing PCR conditions from microdissected formalin-fixed and paraffin-embedded materials. Pathobiology 2000; 68:215-7.
20. Gloghini A, Canal B, Klein U et al. RT-PCR analysis of RNA extracted from Bouin-fixed and paraffin-embedded lymphoid tissues. J Mol Diagn 2004; 6:290-6.
21. Florell SR, Coffin CM, Holden JA et al. Preservation of RNA for functional genomic studies: A multidisciplinary tumor bank protocol. Mod Pathol 2001; 14:116-28.
22. Roos-van Groningen MC, Eikmans M, Baelde HJ et al. Improvement of extraction and processing of RNA from renal biopsies. Kidney Int 2004; 65:97-105.
23. Kunz Jr GM, Chan DW. The use of laser capture microscopy in proteomics research—a review. Dis Markers 2004; 20:155-60.
24. Ehrig T, Abdulkadir SA, Dintzis SM et al. Quantitative amplification of genomic DNA from histological tissue sections after staining with nuclear dyes and laser capture microdissection. J Mol Diagn 2001; 3:22-5.
25. Burgemeister R, Gangnus R, Haar B et al. High quality RNA retrieved from samples obtained by using LMPC (laser microdissection and pressure catapulting) technology. Pathol Res Pract 2003; 199:431-6.
26. Okuducu AF, Janzen V, Hahne JC et al. Influence of histochemical stains on quantitative gene expression analysis after laser-assisted microdissection. Int J Mol Med 2003; 11:449-53.
27. Craven RA, Totty N, Harnden P et al. Laser capture microdissection and two-dimensional polyacrylamide gel electrophoresis: Evaluation of tissue preparation and sample limitations. Am J Pathol 2002; 160:815-22.
28. Fend F, Emmert-Buck MR, Chuaqui R et al. Immuno-LCM: Laser capture microdissection of immunostained frozen sections for mRNA analysis. Am J Pathol 1999; 154:61-6.
29. Fend F, Kremer M, Quintanilla-Martinez L. Laser capture microdissection: Methodical aspects and applications with emphasis on immuno-laser capture microdissection. Pathobiology 2000; 68:209-14.
30. Fink L, Kinfe T, Seeger W et al. Immunostaining for cell picking and real-time mRNA quantitation. Am J Pathol 2000; 157:1459-66.
31. Fink L, Kinfe T, Stein MM et al. Immunostaining and laser-assisted cell picking for mRNA analysis. Lab Invest 2000; 80:327-33.
32. Burbach GJ, Dehn D, Nagel B et al. Laser microdissection of immunolabeled astrocytes allows quantification of astrocytic gene expression. J Neurosci Methods 2004; 138:141-8.

Complementary Techniques:
Validation of Gene Expression Data by Quantitative Real Time PCR

Maurizio Provenzano and Simone Mocellin*

Abstract

Microarray technology can be considered the most powerful tool for screening gene expression profiles of biological samples. After data mining, results need to be validated with highly reliable biotechniques allowing for precise quantitation of transcriptional abundance of identified genes. Quantitative real time PCR (qrt-PCR) technology has recently reached a level of sensitivity, accuracy and practical ease that support its use as a routine bioinstrumentation for gene level measurement. Currently, qrt-PCR is considered by most experts the most appropriate method to confirm or confute microarray-generated data. The knowledge of the biochemical principles underlying qrt-PCR as well as some related technical issues must be beard in mind when using this biotechnology.

PCR-Based Analysis of Gene Quantitation

Polymerase chain reaction (PCR)-based techniques allow us to obtain genetic information through the specific amplification of nucleic acid sequences starting with a very low number of target copies. These reactions are characterized by a logarithmic amplification of the target sequences, i.e., increase of PCR copies followed by a plateau phase showing a rapid decrease to zero of copy number increment per cycle. Accordingly, the amount of specific DNA product at the end of the PCR run bears no correlation to the number of target copies present in the original specimen. However, many applications in medicine or research require quantification of the number of specific targets in the specimen both to study the reaction of the cell or cell population to a stimulus and to compare the gene profile of different samples. Although PCR analysis gives no information on the biologically active products of genes (i.e., proteins), functional genomics studies have demonstrated a tight correlation between the function of a protein and the expression patterns of its gene.[1] This provides a compelling reason for a gene profile based formulation of scientific hypotheses.

The fundamental importance of gene expression quantification methods in basic research, pharmacogenomics and molecular diagnostics continues to direct efforts aimed at improving current methodologies as well as the development of novel technologies. Not all are based on target amplification: the 'Invader' assay is a development of the invasive signal amplification assay that combines two signal amplification reactions in series to generate and amplify a fluorescent signal in the presence of the correct target sequence.[2] However, reverse transcription (RT)-PCR-based assays are currently the most common method for

*Corresponding Author: Simone Mocellin—Department of Oncological and Surgical Sciences, University of Padova, via Giustiniani 2, 35128 Padova, Italy. Email: mocellins@hotmail.com

Microarray Technology and Cancer Gene Profiling, edited by Simone Mocellin.
©2007 Landes Bioscience and Springer Science+Business Media.

characterising or confirming gene expression patterns and comparing gene levels in different sample populations. Serial analysis of gene expression (SAGE) allows for high-throughput gene profiling.[3] However, this technique is cumbersome, time-consuming and requires multiple manipulations of the samples, increasing the risk of carry over contamination. Furthermore, like Northern and Southern blot, it requires large amounts of input mRNA, making impossible the analysis of hypocellular specimens.

Among the most promising innovations applied to conventional RT-PCR protocols is the development of quantitative RT-PCR such as competitive standardized RT-PCR and quantitative real time PCR (qrt-PCR). These technologies present two major advantages: (1) the use of standardised competitor templates or standard curves, which allows comparison between experiments and (2) the use of internal standards, which addresses the issue of variation in template starting amounts and operator loading errors. Competitive RT-PCR is a time-consuming system, which is limited to sets of primers available from one supplier. Furthermore, it does not eliminate the errors associated with individuals carrying out the reactions.

Conceptual simplicity, practical ease and high-throughput capacity[4] have made real-time fluorescence detection assay the most widely used gene quantification method.[5] In the oncology field, qrt-PCR is experiencing a rapid diffusion among investigators because of its potential applicability to a number of researches. Qrt-PCR allows a highly sensitive quantification of DNA and transcriptional gene levels in a few hours with minimal handling of the samples. The recent flood of reports using qrt-PCR in cancer research testifies the transformation of this technology from an experimental tool into the scientific mainstream.

Principles

The concept of "real time" PCR consists of the detection of PCR products as they accumulate.[6] Current qrt-PCR systems are based on a set of probe and primers, which accounts for the high specificity of the technique. The development of fluorogenic probes[7] eliminated the need of post-PCR processing proper of previous systems. Two main techniques are now available, which exploit the extension[8] or annealing[9] phase, respectively, to generate fluorescence emission (Figs. 1, 2, 3). In both cases, the fluorescence signal increases with each PCR amplification cycle. The PCR cycle number at which fluorescence reaches a threshold value of ten times the standard deviation of baseline fluorescence emission is used for quantitative measurement (Fig. 4). This cycle number is called the cycle threshold (Ct) and it is inversely proportional to the starting amount of target genetic material (Fig. 5). By using probes labelled with different fluorochromes characterized by unique emission spectra, more genes can be analysed at the same time within a given sample (multiplex qrt-PCR).[10]

Although qrt-PCR analysis is sometime referred to as absolute gene quantitation, this term can be misleading. In fact, no matter what the source or how carefully it is measured, there is no way to know exactly how many copies of a known template truly exists in a given well of a known sample.[11] A more appropriate term for this method is standard curve-based quantitation, as a standard curve (fivefold or 10-fold serial dilution) of calculated amount of a given gene is used to quantify the gene abundance in a sample of interest.

Since both the amount of genetic material added to each reverse transcription reaction tube (based on waive length absorbance) and its quality (i.e., degradation) are not reliable parameters in order to measure the starting material, the number of copies of an endogenous control gene—generally referred to as housekeeping gene—is also quantified. For each experimental sample the value of both the target and the housekeeping gene are extrapolated from the respective standard curve equation (Fig. 5). The target value is then divided by the endogenous reference value to obtain a normalized target value independent from the amount of starting material. The assumption must be made that the chosen reference gene does not vary in copy number or expression level under different experimental conditions. Only if this assumption holds true, then multiple samples will be completely comparable.

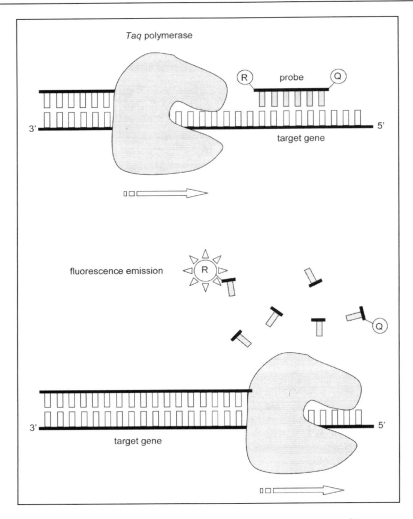

Figure 1. Principles of quantitative real time PCR using fluorogenic probes: scheme of the extension phase method with standard probe. In addition to forward and reverse primers, this system utilizes a probe, which is an oligonucleotide with both a reporter fluorescent dye (R) and a quencher dye (Q) attached at its 5' and 3' end, respectively. During the extension phase, the quencher can only quench the reporter fluorescence when the two dyes are close to each other. This is only the case of an intact probe. In fact, once amplification occurs, the probe is degraded by the 5'-3' exonuclease activity of the *Thermophilus aquaticus (Taq)* DNA polymerase and the fluorescence will be detected by means of a laser integrated in the sequence detector.

Main Issues

Results Normalization

The identification of a valid reference for data normalisation is a crucial issue in qrt-PCR experimental design. Glyceraldehyde-3-phosphate dehydrogenase (GAPDH) is one of the most popular housekeeping genes, although it has been documented that GAPDH mRNA levels are

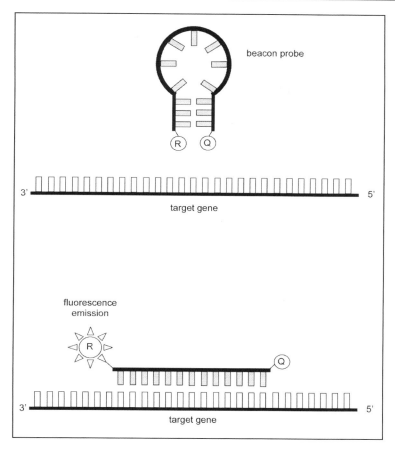

Figure 2. Principles of quantitative real time PCR using fluorogenic probes: scheme of the extension phase method with beacon probe. Molecular beacons are hairpin-shaped molecules with an internally quenched fluorophore whose fluorescence is restored when they bind to a target nucleic acid. They are designed in such a way that the loop portion of the molecule is a probe sequence complementary to a target nucleic acid molecule. The stem is formed by the annealing of complementary arm sequences on the ends of the probe sequence. A fluorescent moiety (R) is attached to the end of one arm and a quenching moiety (Q) is attached to the end of the other arm. The stem keeps these two moieties in close proximity to each other, causing the fluorescence of the fluorophore to be quenched. When the probe encounters a target molecule, the molecular beacon undergoes a spontaneous conformational reorganization that forces the stem apart, and causes the fluorophore and the quencher to move away from each other, leading to the restoration of fluorescence.

not always constant,[12] particularly under same pathological conditions.[13] We and other authors routinely use β-actin as housekeeping gene.[14,15] Even though the issues regarding β-actin gene regulation and pseudogene existence have been raised,[16,17] the consistency of results yielded over time support *ex adjuvantibus* the use of this reference gene. Alternatively, ribosomal RNA, which makes up the bulk of a total RNA sample, is another normaliser that has been proposed,[16] despite reservations concerning its expression levels, transcription by a different RNA polymerase and possible imbalances in rRNA and mRNA fractions between different samples.[18] Other investigators have advocated normalisation to total cellular RNA as the least

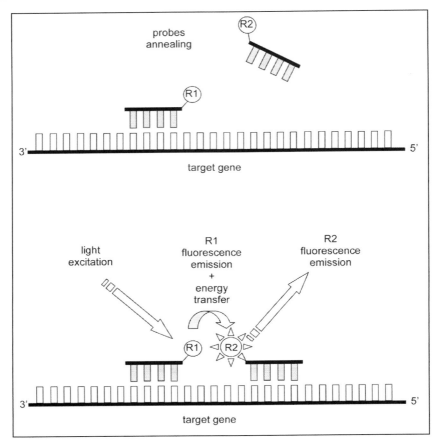

Figure 3. Principles of quantitative real time PCR using fluorogenic probes: scheme of the annealing phase method. In this case, two different probes are used, one carrying a fluorescent reporter at its 3' end (R1), whereas the other carries another fluorescent dye at its 5' end (R2). The sequences of these two oligonucleotides are selected such that they hybridize to the amplified DNA fragment in a head-to-tail arrangement. When the oligonucleotides hybridize in this orientation, the two fluorescence dyes are positioned in close proximity to each other. The first dye (R1) is excited by the filtered light source, and emits a fluorescent light at a slightly longer wavelength. When the two dyes are in close proximity, the energy emitted by R1 excites R2 attached to the second hybridization probe, which subsequently emits fluorescent light at an even longer wavelength. This energy transfer is referred to as FRET (Fluorescence Resonance Energy Transfer). Choosing the appropriate detection channel, the intensity of the light emitted by R2 is filtered and measured.

unreliable method.[19] However, little is known about the total RNA content per cell of different tissues in vivo, or how this might vary between individuals or between normal and tumor tissue. In order to minimize the potential variability characteristic of each single housekeeping gene, some investigators have recently proposed the normalization of qrt-PCR data by geometric averaging of a set of reference genes.[20]

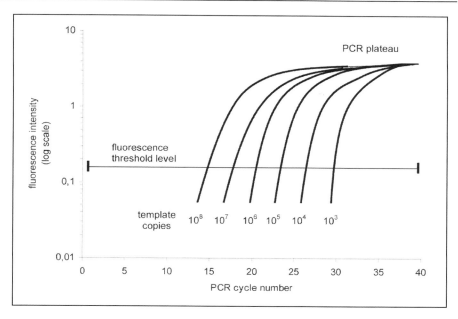

Figure 4. Beta-actin amplification plot illustrating the nomenclature typically used in quantitative real time-PCR experiments. The amplification plot is the plot of fluorescence signal vs PCR cycle number. The signal measured during these PCR cycles is used to plot the threshold. The threshold is calculated as 10 times the standard deviation of the average signal of the baseline fluorescent signal. A fluorescent signal that is detected above the threshold is considered a real signal that can be used to define the threshold cycle (Ct) for a sample. The Ct is defined as the fractional PCR cycle number at which the fluorescent signal is greater than the minimal detection level. The Ct values of different β-actin concentrations are used to generate the standard curve and then calculate the relative equation (Fig. 5).

Messenger RNA Cell Source

When dealing with cell lines or in vitro purified cell populations the issue of gene expression normalization is strictly about the best way to correctly measure gene copy number. Ex vivo samples present an additional problem regarding qrt-PCR data interpretation. In fact, until recently, in vivo RNA extractions and subsequent analyses could be only carried out from whole tissue biopsies with little regard for the different cell types contained within that sample. This inevitably results in the averaging of the expression of different cell types and the expression profile of a specific cell type may be masked, lost or ascribed to and dismissed as illegitimate transcription because of the bulk of the surrounding cells. This is particularly relevant when comparing gene expression profiles between normal and cancer tissue since normal cells adjacent to a tumor may be phenotypically normal, but genotypically abnormal or exhibit altered gene expression profiles due to their proximity to the tumor,[21] and some tumors have significantly larger immune cell infiltrates than others.[22] Recent technology developments might bring a solution to this important issue. In particular, the introduction of laser capture microdissection[23,24] represents a crucial step forward, allowing the extraction of a pure sub-population of cells from heterogeneous in vivo cell samples for detailed molecular analysis.[25] Furthermore, after the introduction of RNA linear amplification,[26] the issue of limited amount of genetic material obtained from tissue microdissection can be easily overcome. Since this RNA method is characterized by a 5'-biased gene amplification, particular attention must be paid to probe/primer design, so that they span the 3'-flank of a given transcript sequence.

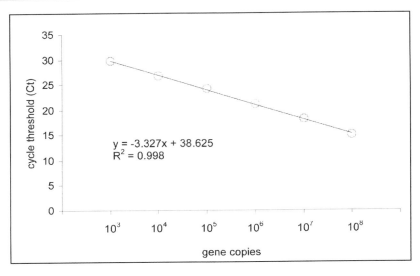

Figure 5. Beta-actin standard curve plot for calculation of PCR efficiency and quantitation. A 10-fold serial dilution of a positive control template is used to generate the standard curve. The resulting Ct values for each input amount of template are plotted as a function of the $\log_{10}$ concentration of input amounts and a linear trend-line is fit to the data. This is done both for optimizing a PCR reaction as measured by the PCR efficiency and for quantitation of unknown samples. The resulting slope of the line fit to the data is used to determine the PCR efficiency as shown in the formula. An ideal slope should be 3.32 for 100% PCR efficiency; in this example it is 97.6%. Optimal standard curves are based on PCR amplification efficiency from 90 to 100% (100% meaning that the amount of template is doubled after each cycle), as demonstrated by the slope of the standard curve equation. Linear regression analysis of all standard curves should show a high correlation (R^2 coefficient ≥ 0.99) to be considered suitable for gene levels quantitative analysis. The function that defines this slope is also used to calculate the amount of unknown samples. Most real-time PCR instruments have software that can automatically compute the amount of template of an unknown sample from a standard curve. However, it can be done manually by putting the observed Ct value for an unknown sample into the formula: (observed Ct - y intercept)/slope.

References

1. Brown PO, Botstein D. Exploring the new world of the genome with DNA microarrays. Nat Genet 1999; 21:33-37.
2. de Arruda M, Lyamichev VI, Eis PS et al. Invader technology for DNA and RNA analysis: Principles and applications. Expert Rev Mol Diagn 2002; 2:487-496.
3. hang L, Zhou W, Velculescu VE et al. Gene expression profiles in normal and cancer cells. Science 1997; 276:1268-1272.
4. Heid CA, Stevens J, Livak KJ et al. Real time quantitative PCR. Genome Res 1996; 6:986-994.
5. Klein D. Quantification using real-time PCR technology: Applications and limitations. Trends Mol Med 2002; 8:257-260.
6. Higuchi R, Dollinger G, Walsh PS et al. Simultaneous amplification and detection of specific DNA sequences. Biotechnology (NY) 1992; 10:413-417.
7. Lee LG, Connell CR, Bloch W et al. Allelic discrimination by nick-translation PCR with fluorogenic probes. Nucleic Acids Res 1993; 21:3761-3766.
8. Lie YS, Petropoulos CJ. Advances in quantitative PCR technology: 5' Nuclease assays. Curr Opin Biotechnol 1998; 9:43-48.
9. Didenko VV. DNA probes using fluorescence resonance energy transfer (FRET): Designs and applications. Biotechniques 2001; 31:1106-1116.
10. Wittwer CT, Herrmann MG, Gundry CN et al. Real-time multiplex PCR assays. Methods 2001; 25:430-442.

11. Ginzinger DG. Gene quantification using real-time quantitative PCR: An emerging technology hits the mainstream. Exp Hematol 2002; 30:503-512.
12. Zhu G, Chang Y, Zuo J et al. Fudenine, a C-terminal truncated rat homologue of mouse prominin, is blood glucose-regulated and can up-regulate the expression of GAPDH. Biochem Biophys Res Commun 2001; 281:951-956.
13. Goidin D, Mamessier A, Staquet MJ et al. Ribosomal 18S RNA prevails over glyceraldehyde-3-phosphate dehydrogenase and beta-actin genes as internal standard for quantitative comparison of mRNA levels in invasive and noninvasive human melanoma cell subpopulations. Anal Biochem 2001; 295:17-21.
14. Kammula US, Marincola FM, Rosenberg SA et al. Real-time quantitative polymerase chain reaction assessment of immune reactivity in melanoma patients after tumor peptide vaccination. J Natl Cancer Inst 2000; 92:1336-1344.
15. Seeger K, Kreuzer KA, Lass U et al. Molecular quantification of response to therapy and remission status in TEL-AML1-positive childhood ALL by real-time reverse transcription polymerase chain reaction. Cancer Res 2001; 61:2517-2522.
16. Selvey S, Thompson EW, Matthaei K et al. Beta-actin—an unsuitable internal control for RT-PCR. Mol Cell Probes 2001; 15:307-311.
17. Raff T, van der Giet M, Endemann D et al. Design and testing of beta-actin primers for RT-PCR that do not co amplify processed pseudogenes. Biotechniques 1997; 23:456-460.
18. Solanas M, Moral R, Escrich E. Unsuitability of using ribosomal RNA as loading control for Northern blot analyses related to the imbalance between messenger and ribosomal RNA content in rat mammary tumors. Anal Biochem 2001; 288:99-102.
19. Bustin SA. Absolute quantification of mRNA using real-time reverse transcription polymerase chain reaction assays. J Mol Endocrinol 2000; 25:169-193.
20. Vandesompele J, De Preter K, Pattyn F et al. Accurate normalization of real-time quantitative RT-PCR data by geometric averaging of multiple internal control genes. Genome Biol 2002; 3:RE-SEARCH0034.
21. Deng G, Lu Y, Zlotnikov G, Thor AD et al. Loss of heterozygosity in normal tissue adjacent to breast carcinomas. Science 1996; 274:2057-2059.
22. Bustin SA, Li SR, Phillips S et al. Expression of HLA class II in colorectal cancer: Evidence for enhanced immunogenicity of microsatellite-instability-positive tumours. Tumour Biol 2001; 22:294-298.
23. Elkahloun AG, Gaudet J, Robinson GS et al. In situ gene expression analysis of cancer using laser capture microdissection, microarrays and real time quantitative PCR. Cancer Biol Ther 2002; 1:354-358.
24. Emmert-Buck MR et al. Laser capture microdissection. Science 1996; 274:998-1001.
25. Walch A, Specht K, Smida J et al. Tissue microdissection techniques in quantitative genome and gene expression analyses. Histochem Cell Biol 2001; 115:269-276.
26. Wang E, Miller LD, Ohnmacht GA et al. High-fidelity mRNA amplification for gene profiling. Nat Biotechnol 2000; 18:457-459.

CHAPTER 6

Microarrays for Cancer Diagnosis and Classification

Ainhoa Perez-Diez,* Andrey Morgun and Natalia Shulzhenko

Abstract

Microarray analysis has yet to be widely accepted for diagnosis and classification of human cancers, despite the exponential increase in microarray studies reported in the literature. Among several methods available, a few refined approaches have evolved for the analysis of microarray data for cancer diagnosis. These include class comparison, class prediction and class discovery. Using as examples some of the major experimental contributions recently provided in the field of both hematological and solid tumors, we discuss the steps required to utilize microarray data to obtain general and reliable gene profiles that could be universally used in clinical laboratories. As we show, microarray technology is not only a new tool for the clinical lab but it can also improve the accuracy of the classical diagnostic techniques by suggesting novel tumor-specific markers. We then highlight the importance of publicly available microarray data and the development of their integrated analysis that may fulfill the promise that this new technology holds for cancer diagnosis and classification.

Introduction

Current cancer classification includes more than 200 types of cancer. For the patient to receive appropriate therapy, the clinician must identify as accurately as possible the cancer type. Although analysis of morphologic characteristics of biopsy specimens is still the standard diagnostic method, it gives very limited information and clearly misses much important tumor aspects such as rate of proliferation, capacity for invasion and metastases, and development of resistance mechanisms to certain treatment agents. To appropriately classify tumor subtypes, therefore, molecular diagnostic methods are needed. The classical molecular methods look for the DNA, RNA or protein of a defined marker that is correlated with a specific type of tumor and may or may not give biological information about cancer generation or progression. However, a major advantage of microarray is the huge amount of molecular information that can be extracted and integrated to find common patterns within a group of samples. As we will show here, microarrays could be used in combination with other diagnostic methods to add more information about the tumor specimen by looking at thousands of genes concurrently. This new method is revolutionizing cancer diagnostics because it not only classifies tumor samples into known and new taxonomic categories, and discovers new diagnostic and therapeutic markers, but it also identifies new subtypes that correlate with treatment outcome.

*Corresponding Author: Ainhoa Perez-Diez—Ghost Lab, Laboratory of Cellular and Molecular Immunology, NIAID, NIH, U.S.A. Email: aperezdiez@niaid.nih.gov

Microarray Technology and Cancer Gene Profiling, edited by Simone Mocellin.
©2007 Landes Bioscience and Springer Science+Business Media.

Revealing Expression Profiles for Cancer Diagnosis and Classification

Data Analysis: Supervised and Unsupervised Methods

Each microarray experiment generates thousands of data points and reports are written in a dense technical jargon. It is easy to feel lost when trying to make sense of it all. For this reason, it is important to clearly define certain technical terms as well as goals of microarray experiments. To understand how microarrays are used, the jargon "class" and, more specifically, "known class" must be first defined. A class refers to any characteristic shared by one group of samples but not other samples: e.g., cancer versus normal tissue, metastatic versus primary tumor, responders to cancer treatment versus nonresponders. A "known class" is any differentiating characteristic that the researcher will use to label the tumor samples under study a priori the data analysis. The two main goals of microarray studies are: (1) to identify molecular signatures associated with known classes, and (2) to discover new classes. To achieve those goals, two different approaches to data analysis are taken, the Supervised method (first goal above) and the Unsupervised method (second goal) (Fig. 1).[1] To read and understand microarray-based studies, knowledge of these different methods, will greatly help to understand the authors' hypothesis and data interpretation.

Supervised methods of analysis are used predominantly to identify the differences at molecular level between known classes (Class Comparison) and to diagnose or "predict" to which class a new tumor sample belongs (Class Prediction). By contrast, in unsupervised methods, the samples are not labeled to belong to different clinicopathologic classes before data analysis (i.e., "unknown class"). When the purpose of the experiment is to test the hypothesis that the samples are composed of different classes, the approach is called Class Discovery. Class Discovery attempts to identify new sub-classes of tumors in cancers where the actual classification needs more definition: for instance, when the classification does not explain the different patient survival after cancer treatment.

In Class Comparison studies, the purpose is to understand the differences in gene expression that might be responsible for the differences between compared classes of tumors and to, perhaps, find hints on the genes that might deserve further study. In cancer diagnosis, however, Class Comparison is usually incorporated into Class Prediction.

Class Prediction studies build a gene "predictor" based on the genes whose expression differs between the different classes of tumors under study. A predictor is a gene expression-based multivariate function that will use the genes identified in Class Comparison to assign new tumor sample(s) into the correct class (Fig. 1). However, this method suffers from one major limitation called over fitting (1). This means that the classification algorithm performs well on the samples from which it was built but poorly on independent samples. Therefore, the validation of the gene predictor is necessary for future clinical applications. The ideal predictor is built with a "training" group of samples and then validated on a "test" group of samples.[2] Moreover, samples in the test and training groups should be preferentially collected and analyzed at different time points in order to ensure independency between them and to validate the predictor in similar conditions as it might be applied in the future. An important caution should be taken into account. Since the samples are a priori classified based on the currently accepted diagnostic tests, which are neither 100% sensitive nor specific, this may decrease the accuracy of the gene predictor by including in the training set a few misclassified samples. Some good examples of this type of study are discussed below.[3-5]

In Class Discovery studies, the samples are grouped depending on their global gene expression without reference to tumor type, grade or any other characteristic. It analyzes the expression of thousands of genes to try to discover new taxonomic groups within the samples (Fig. 1). As an unsupervised method, it will uncover the predominant relationship of the samples' gene signature, which not always corresponds with the potential clinically relevant relationship. Examples of this kind of studies are discussed later in the chapter.[3,5-9]

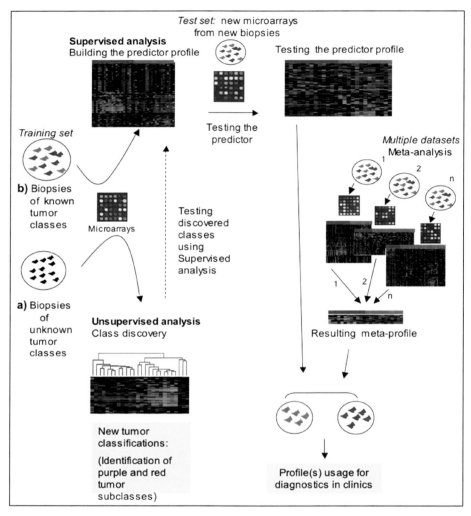

Figure 1. Analysis of microarray data to discover new tumor classification and to build gene predictors for cancer diagnosis. a) For class discovery, biopsies, which we hypothesize belong to different tumor classes (black biopsies), are analyzed by unsupervised methods to see the global similarities and differences between them at the molecular level. In this case, the biopsies formed two main clusters (green and blue) depending on their gene expression, which means that there are indeed 2 different classes within our samples. b) To build a gene predictor profile for cancer diagnosis we analyze samples that belong to the 2 classes we want to distinguish (purple and red). The supervised analysis will give the list of genes that are differentially regulated in one class with respect to the other. This list of genes will form the predictor profile. A new group of samples of known classes (test set) is analyzed to test the validity of the predictor. For this, the gene predictor profile is used to assign test set samples to one of the classes. Gene profiles created in different laboratories can be combined in a meta-profile. Resulting profiles are applied for diagnostics.

Examples from the Literature

Over the last few years, many studies have focused on the classification and diagnosis of cancer using microarray technology. Here, we will discuss a few examples that show how this technique can improve on the information given by classical diagnostic methods. The first three studies are in hematological malignancies, for a more extended review on the microarray advances in this area you can read Eber and Golub,[10] and the next four studies are in solid tumors.

Hematological Malignancies

The initial microarray studies were focused on hematological tumors for two main reasons: (1) purification of certain cell populations from the tumor samples is easy according to cell surface markers (for instance, Alizadeh et al purified chronic lymphocyte leukaemia cells by using CD19, a B-cell marker) or through Ficoll sedimentation to obtain mononuclear cells from peripheral blood or bone marrow specimens[3,5] and (2) wide knowledge of hematopoiesis and its genetic regulation helped to understand the complicated gene expression data generated by microarrays.

Example of Class Prediction

In 1999, a pioneer study analyzed 38 bone marrow samples from acute leukemia patients.[3] Acute leukemia can be divided into two groups: acute myeloid leukemia (AML) and acute lymphoblastic leukemia (ALL). The problem is that for such diagnosis, several diagnostic techniques need to be run because no single one is currently sufficient and even then, the diagnosis is not always correct. The authors used supervised analysis for Class prediction to come up with a list of 50 genes that were differentially expressed between the initial 27 ALL and 11 AML training samples. Then, they apply the predictor of 50 genes to a test set of 34 new leukemia samples independently collected from the training samples. Twenty-nine of the 34 samples that formed the test set were correctly classified, supporting the possibility that in the future gene predictors obtained from larger training set of samples, could be used to supplement existing diagnostic methods. Many of the genes that formed the predictor set encoded for proteins important for cell cycle, cell adhesion, transcription or oncogenes, which could give insights into cancer pathogenesis and pharmacology as well as having diagnostic value. As a second goal of this study, the authors used Class discovery method on the initial 38 leukemia samples to see whether global gene expression analysis could have distinguished between AML and ALL if these two diagnostic classes would not have been known a priori. By using self-organizing maps (SOM), where the user specifies the number of classes to be identified, and setting them in two, 24 of the 25 ALL samples were cluster together in one group and 10 of the 13 AML samples were clustered in the second one. This showed that Class discovery studies are able to uncover diagnostic classes of tumor in cases when morphological or phenotypical tests are not, although biological and clinical information seemed necessary to interpret the results.

Examples of Class Discovery: The Basis for Predicting Prognosis

The next two studies[5,7] are good examples of how Class discovery approach is able to resolve new taxonomic subclasses. The discovery of new classes, when added to clinical information linked to them (as it is survival after treatment), can give very important additional prognostic information.

Alizadeh et al[7] studied large B-cell lymphoma (DLBCL), the most common subtype of nonHodgkin's lymphoma, for which there are not reliable morphological, clinical, immuno-histochemical or genetic diagnostic markers to recognize possible subclasses.[11] By using unsupervised methods for Class discovery on samples from 40 DLBCL patients, the authors were able to distinguish two previously unknown groups of DLBCL. The two groups were called "germinal center B-like DLBCL" and "activated B-like DLBCL" because the main differences between them were genes involved in B-cell activation and in germinal center formation. These two new taxonomic groups are not only biologically relevant, but they also have an important prognostic value, as the authors showed that five years after anthracycline-based chemotherapy treatment, 76% of germinal center B-like DLBCL patients survived, while only 16% of activated B-like DLBCL did.

More recently, Bullinger et al[5] made a larger scale study on 116 samples from adults with AML including 45 with normal karyotype. Even though karyotype abnormalities are the most powerful prognostic factor in AML patients,[12,13] 35% to 50% of patients showing a normal karyotype have an unpredictable prognosis. Class discovery analysis of all the AML samples divided them into new molecular subclasses. Interestingly, the 45 patients with normal karyotype were divided in two groups that were found to have different survival rates. The authors then built a 133 genes predictor that was able to differentiate among patients with normal karyotype into good and poor prognosis. This study was the first one able to do so in AML patients with normal karyotype. Although the initial purpose of this study was the Class discovery of new subtypes of AML, the complementary clinical information on survival rates allowed the additional prognostic value to the new AML classification.

Solid Tumors

Solid tumor biopsies not only contain malignant cells, but may also contain different percentages of fibroblasts, endothelial, and immune cells that will influence the mRNA pool of the sample. Therefore, it was thought that the heterogeneity of cell types within the biopsies would not allow for "clean" cancer specific genetic studies.[14] For this reason, some authors preferred to purify the tumor cells from the biopsy by laser capture microdisection[15] before doing gene expression studies. Some studies have shown, however, that the data obtained from the whole tumor is very similar to the data obtained by laser microdisected tumor cells from the same specimens.[16,17] Besides, nonmalignant cells in the tumor microenvironment may play a role in tumor formation, response to treatment and metastases formation.[18-20] By purifying only malignant cells from the tumor biopsies, not only this information will be lost but it will also increase the cost and time of the procedure, making harder for microarrays to be implemented as a regularly used clinical diagnostic method. The studies below prove that purification of malignant cells might not be necessary to obtain reliable and useful diagnostic information from solid tumors.

Examples of Class Prediction: Improving Treatment Decisions

Gene expression analysis proved able to detect the metastatic potential of primary tumors.[4] In this work, 12 metastatic adenocarcinoma nodules of diverse origin (lung, breast, prostate, colorectal, uterus, and ovary) were compared with 64 primary adenocarcinomas representing the same tumor types from different individuals, forming a training set of 76 samples. The authors found 128 genes differentially expressed between the metastatic and the primary tumors and use these genes to build a predictor that was tested to classify primary tumors of different origins (62 lung adenocarcinomas, 78 primary breast adenocarcinomas, 21 prostate adenocarcinomas, 60 medulloblastomas). They found that all the previous tumors were divided into two classes depending on how similar their molecular profile were to the metastases one. The conclusion of the study is that primary tumors carrying the metastases-like gene expression signature were associated with metastasis and worse clinical outcome. Another interesting feature of this work is that the authors used data developed from different laboratories on different array platforms to test their 128 genes predictor.

In a more recent work that analyzed primary head and neck squamous cell carcinomas (HNSCCs) Roepman et al[9] were able to build a gene predictor that could detect local lymph node metastases using material from primary HNSCCs. The predictor, formed by 102 genes, outperformed current clinical diagnostic methods with an overall predictive accuracy of 86%, while the current diagnostic method had 68%. This improvement in the diagnosis has a lot of relevance for treatment selection and the authors estimated that by using microarrays to diagnose the existence of local metastases, 75% of patients that were really metastasis-free but diagnosed as carrying possible metastases, could have avoided radical neck dissection treatment. This work also presents interesting biological information about the genes differentially expressed between the two classes of primary tumors compared here: those with local metastases and those without local metastases. Interestingly, half of the 102 genes that formed the predictor have unknown role in metastases formation and could give more insights into how this process occurs.

Examples of Class Discovery

As an example of class discovery study, Bittner et al[6] were able to identify previously unrecognized subtypes of cutaneous melanoma by gene expression studies of 31 melanoma biopsies. The authors found a group of 19 melanoma tumors that clustered together showing strong similarities at molecular level. Despite the lack of statistical association of this group of melanoma samples with any clinical variable, they showed that samples within this group had reduced motility and invasiveness in in vitro tests respect to samples that didn't belong to the group. This was a nice attempt to use gene expression profiling for the generation of melanoma taxonomy, however it shows the difficulties of doing so when such taxonomy is not linked to easily detectable clinical differences.

Another Class discovery study[8] was able to differentiate 4 sub-groups of breast tumors: estrogen receptor positive/luminal-like, basal-like, *Erb-B2* positive and normal breast tissue-like, when separating a total of 65 samples according to the expression of 496 genes. Interestingly, the four subtypes were not visible in a first analysis of their data, when they looked at a larger number of genes. The reason for this was the use of different gene selection criteria. The first list of 1,753 genes was based on the assumption that all the samples were independent between each other. However, there were 20 pair-wise comparisons of the same tumors before and after chemotherapy. When trying to group the 65 samples according to their global gene expression, the similarities between the samples coming from the same tumor overcame the similarities between the samples coming from a hypothetical same tumor subtype. Results from this first analysis showed the need to treat pair wise samples as if they belonged to the same tumor subtype and look for other samples that had similar gene expression. These biological criteria were used to create a second list of 496 genes that revealed the 4 breast cancer subtypes; this is an example of how biologist and statistician must work together to resolve the intricacy of gene expression analysis. This new classification of breast tumors has been supported by a follow up study.[21]

Overall, microarrays have a remarkable potential as a new diagnostic tool in oncology showing substantial improvements over conventional diagnostic and classification criteria for many different types of tumors. Better diagnosis will improve the decision making process to choose the right treatment. Better classification, when combined with treatment response data, will improve cancer prognosis.

Using Expression Profiles in the Clinic

How to Apply a Published Microarray Class Predictor to Classify New Samples

Despite great advances in discovering cancer molecular profiles, the proper application of microarray technology to routine clinical diagnostics is still unresolved. One key limitation is that an individual tumor cannot be classified independently. It needs to be compared to other samples or "standards", whose classification is known, and which are analyzed under the same conditions as the individual tumor. For this, some points appear to be critical. First, if the predictor was created in the same lab as the sample of interest being analyzed, the sample preparation, array set up, reference sample (for two-color design), slide processing and analysis should be exactly the same as for the original set. The major limitation here might be the availability of the same reference sample. When using one-color design, it is not necessary to use reference sample for hybridization, but all other cautions are essential for the correct classification. Second, if one wants to apply predictor genes discovered in another lab, then the task is more complex. In order to obtain comparable results, usage of the originally established protocol is essential. Recently the question of interlaboratory comparability was addressed for microarray data on human tumor specimens.[22] This work showed that, under similar technical conditions, a high correlation between gene expressions in repeated samples could be obtained regardless of the laboratory in which the experiments were done. However, even when using the same protocol and microarray platform, it is still necessary to analyze a set of known samples together with the unknown one/s. Furthermore, a large number of samples from several independent datasets are required to guarantee the applicability of the validated profiles.[23] Although demanding, the application of a molecular profile (previously described in one laboratory) by a second laboratory with a slightly different framework may represent an important benefit. In fact, it helps to define how general or specific to certain situation/s the profile is. For example, a set of 231 genes was described by van't Veer et al[24] as discriminating for prognosis in node-negative untreated breast cancer patients. However, a different laboratory found that a subset of 93 genes, out of the 231 genes forming the predictor, was valid to make the same discrimination even in a more heterogeneous population of node-positive/negative patients treated with adjuvant therapy.[25]

Translation of microarray profiles into clinical practice is already beginning in some academic centers in the Netherlands and United States and profiles that have been validated in retrospective studies are now being applied in prospective clinical trials.[26]

How to Select Biomarkers from a Microarray Class Predictor

Another way to explore genome-wide expression data for cancer diagnosis is to translate this information into surrogate molecular markers (Fig. 2). There are at least two important advantages for doing this. First, they can be measured by relatively cheap and widely used clinical methods such as RT-PCR, ELISA and immunohistochemistry. Second, they can be detected in serum or other body fluids permitting the establishment of noninvasive diagnostic test, which is very important especially in the cases of cancers with more difficult access for diagnostic biopsy (e.g., lung, ovary, pancreas). Usually, the biomarkers will be chosen from the list of genes that form a predictor. But genes that, when combined, were good predicting the class to which a new sample belongs are not necessary good biomarkers when used alone or combined with just a few other genes. Microarray predictors usually consist of tens or hundreds of molecules. Therefore, two of the main questions for translation of microarray classifiers into diagnostic markers are: first, which genes should be selected from microarray profiles and second, how to select the minimum number of these genes sufficient for good diagnostic classification. Although several statistical procedures were suggested for this purpose,[27,28] currently there is no consensus about the best one. Apparently, the use of multiple algorithms increases the confidence and validity of the selected genes.[28]

At the moment, real time RT-PCR is the most widely used technique for validation of microarray results as well as for attempting to substitute the microarray profiles for diagnostic markers. It is important to remember that, despite its similarity to microarray measurement, RT-PCR could give slightly different results. A factor that greatly contributes to the difference is the normalization procedure, which is much more precise in microarrays than in RT-PCR. In fact, microarrays generally use global normalization including all genes expressed by the sample (usually a few thousands) since the majority of the genes don't show significant expression variation across all the samples. Consequently, the normalization is not influenced as much (as it is in RT-PCR) when one or a few control (or housekeeping) genes don't behave as such and show variation on their expression among the samples.

Gordon and colleagues[29] proposed an interesting solution in the form of a ratio-based method of samples classification that circumvents this problem. First, ratios between genes showing opposite expressions in the clinical groups of samples are calculated. Then, samples are assigned to one of the groups accordingly to the value of the ratio. The authors used this approach in two studies. In the first one,[29] malignant pleural mesothelioma and adenocarcinoma of the lung were differentially diagnosed by means of eight genes. Five were up-regulated and three were down-regulated in mesothelioma respect to adenocarcinoma giving, therefore,

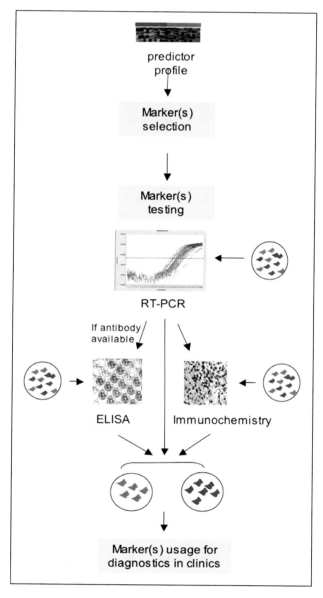

Figure 2. Discovering and testing diagnostic markers. Markers can be selected from the gene predictor profile illustrated in Figure 1. Selected markers are measured by quantitative RT-PCR in a test set of samples to check assignments of samples to the classes. If there is antibody available for the selected marker, it could also be tested by ELISA and/or immunochemistry. Markers with good performance are applied for diagnostics.

15 ratios. Any individual ratio had at least 90% of accuracy discriminating the tumor samples and they reached 99% when 3 random ratios were combined. In the second one,[30] the same authors selected some genes from the published microarray data in prostate cancers,[31,32]

created the optimal ratio-based test and examined it using RT-PCR in an additional cohort of cancer and normal tissue. A 3-ratio test using 4 genes was 90% accurate distinguishing normal prostate and cancer samples. Thus, the most important feature of this solution is that using gene expression ratios it is possible to avoid the selection of "right" housekeeping genes and the normalization process for assignment of samples to classes.

However, even using conventional normalization of RT-PCR results, the microarray results can be translated into RT-PCR diagnostic profiles. In fact, Lossos and colleagues[33] studied by RT-PCR 36 genes whose expression had been reported to predict survival in diffuse large-B-cell lymphoma based on microarray data. Six genes that were among the strongest predictors entered the multivariate model and were able to distinguish different survival groups.

Similarly, a diagnostic discrimination between benign and malignant esophageal tissue was proposed using the expression of the most informative genes selected from microarrays and further evaluated by RT-PCR.[34] In this study, logistic regression and linear discriminant analysis were applied for the selection of clinically useful gene-classifiers. Continuing in the same field of gastrointestinal oncology and following up microarray experiments, Mori et al[35] found highly specific markers that detected minuscule amounts of cancer cells in cytology-negative peritoneal washings by RT-PCR. Importantly, they prospectively identified a proportion of patients with minimal residual disease that could not be diagnosed and treated otherwise.

Because RT-PCR can easily and fast detect mRNA levels of considerably many genes, and it does not depend on availability of specific reagents (like antibodies), it is the most rapid translation method of microarray observations into clinical practice. ELISA and immunohistochemistry, however, detect proteins in quantitative or semi-quantitative manner. Therefore, these two methods require a more complex procedure for marker selection and validation, since not only the mRNA expression needs to be validated but also the level of the corresponding protein in tissue and or serum.

To increase a chance that marker candidates selected from large scale gene expression data will pass all rigorous validation requirements, results of microarrays from different studies could be screened. An example of a tissue marker discovered using data from several microarray datasets is alpha-methylacyl CoA racemase (AMACR).[36] AMACR was selected using 4 independent datasets where the gene was over-expressed in prostate cancer comparing to benign prostate tissue. During validation in an independent set of samples, the same results were obtained when measuring mRNA and protein expression using RT-PCR and immunoblot, respectively. Then immunohistochemistry on tissue array was applied to analyze a large number of samples and evaluate clinical utility of AMACR. Interestingly, AMACR immunostaining showed not only good sensitivity (97%) and specificity (100%) for prostate cancer in the whole sample population, but it performed well also in diagnostically challenging cases that needed additional expert pathological review.

Similarly, the proteins villin and moesin were found to be tissue biomarkers that successfully distinguished between colon and ovarian adenocarcinomas.[37] To do so, the authors measured gene expression and protein levels in tumor cell lines. As a result of these experiments and also based on antibody availability, villin and moesin were selected as candidates for colorectal adenocarcinoma and ovarian adenocarcinoma, respectively. Then, after sequence verification, and corroboration of mRNA expression using Affimetrix array, they validated the protein levels. This was done by protein lysate microarrays followed by immunohistochemistry on tissue microarray where the authors obtained high sensitivity and specificity for both markers. This and the AMACR studies represent good examples on how a multi-step approach including genomic, proteomic, and tissue array profiling, results in selection of very few but efficient diagnostic tissue markers.

From a diagnostic point of view, serum cancer markers are even more important than tissue markers because of their ease of procurement for large screenings for early cancer diagnosis. However, the search for serum markers is the more challenging. In fact, a candidate for serum marker, selected from gene expression profiles, should not only be over-expressed locally in the cancer microenvironment, but also codes for a protein that is secreted to the periphery in sufficient levels to be detected in blood. In this situation, bioinformatics tools like Gene Ontologies are helpful to choose genes with the characteristics of interest (e.g., secreted molecule) among the huge amount of differentially expressed genes.

Ovarian cancer is a good example of discovery of serum markers. This type of cancer is usually diagnosed in advanced stage, when only about 28% of the patients survive 5 years.[38] In a series of studies, three serum diagnostic candidates (prostatin, osteopontin and creatine kinase B) were evaluated.[37-39] By microarrays, the authors found these three proteins (among many others) over-expressed in ovarian tumor versus normal cell lines and the three markers were selected based on antibodies availability. After corroboration of the results by real time RT-PCR and immunohistochemistry, the authors screened sera from patients with ovarian cancer, benign disease, and healthy controls by ELISA. The results showed a strong association between increased levels of the markers and ovarian cancer. Perhaps future works combining all three markers and in a larger sample setting will show how useful these three markers could be in diagnostic screening of ovarian cancer.

Overall, microarray expression profiles are an excellent source of useful markers, which will allow the diagnosis of different tumors by conventional techniques in clinical laboratories.

Perspective

As the mass of transcriptome data for cancer diagnosis/classification continues to grow and each single study may have a limited power and validity, there is the need for combined analysis of publicly available data. To reach this goal, every new publication in this field is required to follow the MIAME (Minimum Information About a Microarray Experiment) guidelines (described in: http://www.mged.org/Workgroups/MIAME/miame_checklist.html) and to deposit its microarray data to an open database. For this purpose, two open databases are most commonly used: Gene Expression Omnibus (http://www.ncbi.nlm.nih.gov/geo/) and Array Express, (http://www.ebi.ac.uk/arrayexpress/). Using this tool, some groups of researchers tried to join data from different microarray works, either to reveal new expression profiles or to select markers for diagnostic assessment by other than microarray techniques.[40-42] Recently, Rhodes and colleagues[41] addressed the question of microarray meta-analysis (i.e., combined analysis of the results of different microarray studies) (Fig. 1) in order to identify common gene expression signatures of human cancers. Contrary to the other studies focused on a single tissue type and model, they collected and analyzed data from more that 3,700 cancer samples representing more than 10 tissue types. A common transcriptional profile ("meta-profile") universally activated across most cancer types compared to normal tissue was detected. In addition, more aggressive, undifferentiated cancers showed a distinct meta-signature. This work identified common features of neoplastic transformation and progression and it is a tool for searching potential universal diagnostic markers.

To reach its full potential in cancer diagnosis and classification microarray technology needs improvement of its ancillary technologies such as development of new microarray platforms, statistics and software for analysis and data mining. This will not only simplify technical and analytical procedures but will also make them more precise and cheaper. In addition, inter-laboratory cooperation for ongoing meta-profiles will help produce standardized diagnostic methods utilizing microarrays.

In conclusion, microarrays are beginning to take an important place in clinical oncology practice. Although the main potential success of microarrays is related to evaluation of patients' prognosis, microarrays also improve current clinical diagnostics, discover new diagnostic markers and identify new taxonomic classes of tumors.

Acknowledgements

We want to thank Brandon Reines for critically reading this chapter.

References

1. Simon R, Radmacher MD, Dobbin K et al. Pitfalls in the use of DNA microarray data for diagnostic and prognostic classification. J Natl Cancer Inst 2003; 95:14-18.
2. Ntzani EE, Ioannidis JP. Predictive ability of DNA microarrays for cancer outcomes and correlates: An empirical assessment. Lancet 2003; 362:1439-1444
3. Golub TR, Slonim DK, Tamayo P et al. Molecular classification of cancer: Class discovery and class prediction by gene expression monitoring. Science 1999; 286:531-537.
4. Ramaswamy S, Ross KN, Lander ES et al. A molecular signature of metastasis in primary solid tumors. Nat Genetics 2003; 33:49-54
5. Bullinger L, Dohner K, Bair E et al. Use of gene-expression profiling to identify prognostic subclasses in adult acute myeloid leukemia. N Engl J Med 2004; 350:1605-1616
6. Bittner M, Meltzer P, Chen Y et al. Molecular classification of cutaneous malignant melanoma by gene expression profiling. Nature 2000; 406:536-540.
7. Alizadeh AA, Eisen MB, Davis RE et al. Distinct types of diffuse large B-cell lymphoma identified by gene expression profiling. Nature 2000; 403:503-511.
8. Perou CM, Sorlie T, Eisen MB et al. Molecular portraits of human breast tumours. Nature 2000; 406:747-752
9. Roepman P, Wessels LF, Kettelarij N et al. An expression profile for diagnosis of lymph node metastases from primary head and neck squamous cell carcinomas. Nat Genet 2005; 37:182-186.
10. Ebert BL, Golub TR. Genomic approaches to hematologic malignancies. Blood 2004; 104:923-932.
11. Harris NL, Jaffe ES, Diebold J et al. World Health Organization classification of neoplastic diseases of the hematopoietic and lymphoid tissues: Report of the Clinical Advisory Committee meeting. J Clin Oncol 1999; 12:3835-3849.
12. Grimwade D, Walker H, Oliver F et al. The importance of diagnostic cytogenetics on outcome in AML: Analysis of 1,612 patients entered into the MRC AML 10 trial. The Medical Research Council Adult and Children's Leukaemia Working Parties. Blood 1998; 92:2322-2333.
13. Bloomfield CD, Lawrence D, Byrd JC et al. Frequency of prolonged remission duration after high-dose cytarabine intensification in acute myeloid leukemia varies by cytogenetic subtype. Cancer Res 1998; 58:4173-4179.
14. Player A, Barrett JC, Kawasaki ES. Laser capture microdissection, microarrays and the precise definition of a cancer cell. Expert Rev Mol Diagn 2004; 4:831-840.
15. Ohyama H, Zhang X, Kohno Y et al. Laser capture microdissection-generated target sample for high-density oligonucleotide array hybridization. Biotechniques 2000; 29:530-536.
16. Ernst T, Hergenhahn M, Kenzelmann M et al. Decrease and gain of gene expression are equally discriminatory markers for prostate carcinoma: A gene expression analysis on total and microdissected prostate tissue. Am J Pathol 2002; 160:2169-2180.
17. Sanchez-Carbayo M, Saint F, Lozano JJ et al. Comparison of gene expression profiles in laser-microdissected, nonembedded, and OCT-embedded tumor samples by oligonucleotide microarray analysis. Clin Chem 2003; 49:2096-2100.
18. Dorudi S, Hart IR. Mechanisms underlying invasion and metastasis. Curr Opin Oncol 1993; 5:130-135.
19. Basset P, Okada A, Chenard MP et al. Matrix metalloproteinases as stromal effectors of human carcinoma progression: Therapeutic implications. Matrix Biol 1997; 15:535-541.
20. Chung LW, Baseman A, Assikis V et al. Molecular insights into prostate cancer progression: The missing link of tumor microenvironment. J Urol 2005; 173:10-20.
21. Sorlie T, Tibshirani R, Parker J et al. Repeated observation of breast tumor subtypes in independent gene expression data sets. Proc Natl Acad Sci USA 2003; 100:8418-8423.
22. Dobbin KK, Beer DG, Meyerson M et al. Interlaboratory comparability study of cancer gene expression analysis using oligonucleotide microarrays. Clin Cancer Res 2005; 11:565-572.
23. Michiels S, Koscielny S, Hill C. Prediction of cancer outcome with microarrays: A multiple random validation strategy. Lancet 2005; 365:488-492.
24. van 't Veer LJ, Dai H, van de Vijver MJ et al. Gene expression profiling predicts clinical outcome of breast cancer. Nature 2002; 415:530-536.
25. Sotiriou C, Neo SY, McShane LM et al. Breast cancer classification and prognosis based on gene expression profiles from a population-based study. Proc Natl Acad Sci USA 2003; 100:10393-10398.
26. Kallioniemi O. Medicine: Profile of a tumour. Nature 2004; 428:379-382.
27. Xiong M, Li W, Zhao J et al. Feature (gene) selection in gene expression-based tumor classification. Mol Genet Metab 2001; 73:239-247.
28. Fu LM, Fu-Liu CS. Multi-class cancer subtype classification based on gene expression signatures with reliability analysis. FEBS Lett 2004; 561:186-190.

29. Gordon GJ, Jensen RV, Hsiao LL et al. Translation of microarray data into clinically relevant cancer diagnostic tests using gene expression ratios in lung cancer and mesothelioma. Cancer Res 2002; 62:4963-4967.
30. Bueno R, Loughlin KR, Powell MH et al. A diagnostic test for prostate cancer from gene expression profiling data. J Urol 2004; 171:903-906.
31. Dhanasekaran SM, Barrette TR, Ghosh D et al. Delineation of prognostic biomarkers in prostate cancer. Nature 2001; 412:822-826.
32. Welsh JB, Sapinoso LM, Su AI et al. Analysis of gene expression identifies candidate markers and pharmacological targets in prostate cancer. Cancer Res 2001; 61:5974-5978.
33. Lossos IS, Czerwinski DK, Alizadeh AA et al. Prediction of survival in diffuse large-B-cell lymphoma based on the expression of six genes. N Engl J Med 2004; 350:1828-1837.
34. Brabender J, Marjoram P, Salonga D et al. A multigene expression panel for the molecular diagnosis of Barrett's esophagus and Barrett's adenocarcinoma of the esophagus. Oncogene 2004; 23:4780-4788.
35. Mori K, Aoyagi K, Ueda T et al. Highly specific marker genes for detecting minimal gastric cancer cells in cytology negative peritoneal washings. Biochem Biophys Res Commun 2004; 313:931-937.
36. Rubin MA, Zhou M, Dhanasekaran SM et al. alpha-Methylacyl coenzyme A racemase as a tissue biomarker for prostate cancer. JAMA 2002; 287:1662-70.
37. Nishizuka S, Chen ST, Gwadry FG et al. Diagnostic markers that distinguish colon and ovarian adenocarcinomas: Identification by genomic, proteomic, and tissue array profiling. Cancer Res 2003; 63:5243-50.
38. Huddleston HG, Wong KK, Welch WR et al. Clinical applications of microarray technology: Creatine kinase B is an up-regulated gene in epithelial ovarian cancer and shows promise as a serum marker. Gynecol Oncol 2005; 96:77-83.
39. Mok SC, Chao J, Skates S et al. Prostasin, a potential serum marker for ovarian cancer: Identification through microarray technology. J Natl Cancer Inst 2001; 93:1458-1464.
40. Kim JH, Skates SJ, Uede T et al. Osteopontin as a potential diagnostic biomarker for ovarian cancer. JAMA 2002; 287:1671-9.
41. Rhodes DR, Yu J, Shanker K et al. Large-scale meta-analysis of cancer microarray data identifies common transcriptional profiles of neoplastic transformation and progression Proc Natl Acad Sci USA 2004; 101:9309-9314.
42. Choi JK, Choi JY, Kim DG et al. Integrative analysis of multiple gene expression profiles applied to liver cancer study. FEBS Lett 2004; 565:93-100.

CHAPTER 7

Gene Profiling for the Prediction of Tumor Response to Treatment:
The Case of Immunotherapy

Vladia Monsurrò and Francesco M. Marincola*

Although anticancer immune responses can occur, the biological mechanisms responsible for them remain largely unexplained. Immunologists have extensively studied specific interactions between immune and cancer cells and have identified cofactors that may modulate the effectiveness of such interactions. In particular, as a result of the increasing molecular understanding of the basis for tumor/host interactions, their complexity has become manifest, leading to the conclusion that no single mechanism can model in humans the phenomenon of tumor rejection. It is likely that, due to human and disease heterogeneity, distinct trails lead to a final common pathway responsible for immune-mediated tumor regression. The synergy of the innate and adaptive immune response is likely to be required for successful tumor rejection. These two systems may act by enhancing and remodeling each of the functions by being recruited and activated at the tumor site by molecules with immune modulatory properties produced in the tumor micro-environment by cancer or tumor-associated normal cells. Such complexity could only be recently appreciated in its extent by high-throughput tools capable of providing a global view of biological processes as they occur. In this chapter, we will present selected examples of high-throughput gene expression profiling that may contribute to the understanding of anticancer immune responses.

By following the simplified model of tumor-specific immunization, it has become apparent that factors other than direct T-cell/tumor cell interactions need to be considered when studying the mechanisms leading to immune rejection of cancer. The genetic background of individual patients may affect the immune response. It is becoming increasingly recognized that polymorphism in humans is not limited to genes associated with antigen presentation.[1] In addition, the biological make up of individual tumors may affect T-cell function through pathways independent of HLA/epitope T-cell receptor engagement.[2,3] To obtain a global view of this complexity encompassing human and tumor heterogeneity, a broader approach to the study of tumor immunology is needed. Tools that allow a comprehensive view of tumor/host interactions will be necessary to identify the biological requirements for tumor rejection.[4]

Experimental Models, Human Polymorphisms and Cancer Heterogeneity

Human polymorphisms are particularly frequent in genes associated with immune function. This is likely the result of an evolutionary adaptation of the organism to an ever-changing

*Corresponding Author: Francesco M. Marincola—Department of Transfusion Medicine, Clinical Center, National Institutes of Health, Immunogenetics Section, 9000 Rockville Pike Bethesda, Maryland 20892 U.S.A. Email: FMarincola@cc.nih.gov

Microarray Technology and Cancer Gene Profiling, edited by Simone Mocellin.
©2007 Landes Bioscience and Springer Science+Business Media.

environment.[1] On the other hand, human cancers are shaped and reshaped during their natural history by the incremental collection of epigenetic changes that deviate from the normal cell behavior constrained by laws of development which prepares them to a regulated social life within an organism by controlling growth and differentiation. By contrast, cancers represent a random convergence toward a selfish cell phenotype that has the only goal of self perpetuation at the expense of the host. As a consequence, the study of tumor immunology in humans represents a complex field merging the intricacy of human immunology with the chaotic pattern of cancer biology. To simplify and control the variables related to the study of tumor/host interactions, scientists have created experimental models that bypass such complexity by inbreeding animals (eliminate differences related to genetic background) and standardizing cancers (eliminate the randomness of cancer cell phenotypes). These strategies provided efficient tools for testing basic immunological concepts;[5-10] however, they missed the essence of human disease.[11] In addition, complexity may prove useful if common patterns associated to the occurrence of a biological process could be identified.[12-15]

While technologies are now available for the study of human disease in its complexity collecting information about thousands of variables at the time,[12,16] the big challenge remains of controlling the amount and quality of clinical material available to study. Special strategies should be implemented to optimize the information obtainable from samples of blood, tumor or other tissues. In addition, as tissues and tumors cannot be as easily removed for experimental purposes from humans as in animals, strategies need to be applied that allow serial sampling of relevant material at different time points without compromising the patient's status. Fine needle aspirates (FNA) allow following the natural history of cancer or its response to therapy with minimal invasiveness and discomfort.[17] In this fashion, the evolution of tumor biology can be followed serially during a given treatment to test its mechanism of action. In addition, samples can be obtained before a given treatment is administered, while leaving the tumor deposit in place to directly compare the biological profile of individual lesions with their survival within the body.

Gene Profiling and T-Cell Phenotypes

Several studies reported that epitope-specific immunization induces tumor antigen (TA)-specific CD8[+] T-cells capable of recognizing human leukocyte antigen (HLA)-matched tumor cells.[18-25] However, with few exceptions,[24] these immune responses are not associated with tumor regression. Among various reasons, CD8[+] T-cells number may not be sufficient to overwhelm a large tumor bulk, their status of differentiation or activation may not be suitable for tumor destruction or they may not localize in the target organ. Some investigators[26,27] suggest that T-cell function rapidly evolves in time after antigen exposure through a continuum that spans beyond the rigid dichotomy of memory versus effector phenotype. These authors followed the transcriptional profile of CD8[+] T-cells following time-limited exposure to antigen in a transgenic mouse model. P14 transgenic mice that harbor P14 CD8[+] T-cells expressing a TCR that recognizes the GP33-41 epitope of the lymphocytic choriomeningitis virus (LCMV) protein were exposed to LCMV infection and the antigen-specific CD8[+] T-cells were harvested 8 and 40 days after. The T-cells rapidly expanded and displayed a broad array of effector functions including cytotoxic potential during the first week, but these functions rapidly regressed in the following contraction phase lasting for a few weeks when T-cells maintained ability to recognize target and express cytokines upon reexposure but lost a large array of cytotoxic and other effector functions.

This model applies well to epitope-specific immunization, which also provides time-limited exposure to TA occurring at intervals with each vaccination, followed by a rest interval generally ranging between 2 to 4 weeks. At the functional genomics level, in the mouse model, global transcript analysis demonstrated that CD8[+] positive cells have a distinct phenotype at different time points from antigen exposure, which can be correlated to functional parameters.[27] During the effector phase that peaks at approximately 8 days, CD8[+] T-cells are cytotoxic ex vivo, can respond to cognate stimulation with production of interferon (IFN)γ and have a genetic profile enriched with the expression of effector/activated T-cell genes including granzyme-A and -B, perforin and FAS ligand. Subsequently, in the contraction phase which ends with a memory phenotype approximately 40 days after antigen exposure, CD8$^+$ T-cells that can still respond to cognate stimulation with IFNγ production lose the ability to kill target cells because of the loss of expression of most genes associated with T-cell effector function. This model of T-cell activation/differentiation seems to better explain experimental observations related to immunization-induced T-cells.[26] In fact, immunization induced T-cells retain an effector phenotype according to commonly used markers (CD27 negative, CCR7 negative, CD45RA^{high}) and can also respond to cognate stimulation with IFNγ secretion, but they do not express perforin and cannot exert cytotoxic functions.[28,29] In our laboratory vaccine-specific CD8$^+$ T-cells were successfully separated using magnetic beads and tetrameric HLA/epitope complex (tHLA) staining; their mRNA was linearly amplified and utilized for microarray analysis.[18,30,31] This work demonstrated that the transcriptional profile of circulating CD8$^+$ T-cells approximates that of memory cells with a relative down-regulation of the expression of genes associated with cytotoxic and other effector functions similar to that observed in the contraction phase in the transgenic mouse model.[18] This observation may explain why the frequency of tHLA-staining, epitope-specific T-cells observed in the peripheral circulation does not correlate with tumor rejection, as these T-cells may be depleted of true effector function.[3]

Interactions between Tumor Cells and TA-Specific T-Cells

Available evidence suggests that circulating vaccine-induced T-cells reach the tumor site and interact with tumor cells.[33] The mRNA level of various cytokines supposedly produced by T-cells was measured before and during immunization by quantitative real-time polymerase chain reaction (qrt-PCR). The genetic profile of individual lesions was followed by serial FNA. This analysis demonstrated that the presence of immunization-induced T-cells in the circulation correlates with increments in cytokine transcription (in particular IFNγ) during immunization. In addition, increased mRNA levels correlated with expression of the antigen targeted by immunization and the localization of tHLA-staining, immunization-specific T-cells intra-tumorally.[33] However, this interaction between immunization-induced T-cells and tumor cells was not sufficient to induce tumor regression, as we could follow the growth of all lesions during treatment. Earlier studies had also shown that intra-tumoral localization of TA-specific T-cells is necessary, but not sufficient for tumor regression. The natural presence of tumor-infiltrating lymphocytes (TIL) in melanoma lesions provides the best evidence that TA-specific CD8$^+$ T-cells populate the tumor microenvironment and yet they are not sufficient to cause tumor regression.[34] In addition, an increased frequency of TA-specific, immunization induced T-cells can be demonstrated during vaccination. Yet, this is not associated with tumor regression.[35] Finally, the adoptive transfer of in vitro-expanded TIL labeled with radioactive.[111] It clearly demonstrated that TIL localization is necessary but not sufficient for tumor regression. TILs localization was observed in all the lesions that responded to therapy, but not all the lesions in which TIL localization was observed responded to treatment.[36]

We hypothesize that TA-specific T-cells may populate the tumor micro-environment naturally or reach it in response to immunization, but in most cases they are not exposed in this effector phase to sufficient stimulation/costimulation for their activation into full effector cells. Tumor cells may lack sufficient antigen presentation, or the tumor micro-environment may lack sufficient costimulatory properties.[9] We favor the second hypothesis, as we have never been able to accumulate evidence that lack of antigen stimulation is a primary reason for tumor unresponsiveness. A recent study, in which the transcriptional profile of tumor lesions was assessed before and during therapy, demonstrated that when lesions do not respond to therapy, no changes can be identified in the expression of the TA targeted by the vaccine.[37] In addition, the level of expression of the TA targeted by the vaccine was not a predictor of responsiveness.[37]

As this study was carried out in lesions that expressed the HLA associated with the immunization, HLA loss could also be excluded as responsible for the clinical outcome. In addition, lack of response was associated with a 'silent' genetic profile characterized by no significant differences in global gene expression between treatment and pretreatment samples.[38] Interestingly, while TA expression was not predictive of response, loss of TA expression was consistently observed during therapy in lesions destined to regress.[37] Loss of TA expression preceded clearance of tumor cell during response, as the expression of other TAs irrelevant to the immunization remained stable and cytological analysis confirmed the presence of tumor cells. Thus, it is likely that TA-specific T-cells induced by immunization reach the tumor site, interact with tumor cells and are exposed to antigen recall, but a secondary costimulation is lacking to further expand their number in vivo and activate their effector function.[3]

The Tumor Microenvironment

The tumor microenvironment is complex, heterogeneous and ever changing in adaptation to immune pressure, response to therapy or simply as a consequence of the genetic instability of cancer cells.[3] Therefore, oversimplifications of its biology distort by definition its essence. It is not useful to focus on one gene or gene product such as interleukin (IL)-10 or Fox-P3 and pretend to explain the behavior of human tumors. More attention should be put into the appreciation of tumor complexity during the monitoring of anticancer immune responses. Most studies, however, stay away from the analysis of the tumor microenvironment because of the difficulty to perform repeated biopsies in humans. Yet, tools are available that provide data that could complement information readily obtained by the serial sampling of blood cells. We have shown that serial analysis of tumor aspirates by FNA can be easily performed and can be applied for genetic profiling.[17,38] This strategy allows direct correlation of experimental observations with clinical parameters. In addition, the same approach can be used to study the mechanism of actions of therapeutic agents, by comparing the expression profile of tumor lesions biopsied before and during therapy.

Influence of Genetic Background and Cancer Heterogeneity on Immune Responsiveness

The quest for clinically relevant biomarkers is taking priority in modern research. In the context of tumor immunology, prediction of immune responsiveness could spare an unnecessary therapy to a patient with an expectedly short life span. In addition, understanding of the biological processes responsible for the immune response could lead to better therapy designs. Thus, it behooves us to focus in strategies to identify predictors of immune responsiveness. To follow an orderly pursuit, immune responsiveness may be predominantly dictated by two fundamental biological components: the genetic background of the patient and/or the biology of individual tumors. The genetic background of patients has not been extensively scrutinized as a predictor of immune responsiveness particularly in the context of TA-specific immunization.[1] The HLA phenotype of the patient is a logical genetic marker that may affect immune responsiveness since HLA molecules modulate the specificity of the antigen presented on the surface of cancer cells.[39] The search for correlations between individual HLA alleles or extended haplotypes and treatment outcome or survival yielded relatively unfruitful, conflicting and mostly inconclusive information.[40-42] Associations have been described between polymorphisms of the *IL-10* gene which are responsible for the differential expression of this cytokine. Polymorphisms of the IL-10 genes appear to be associated with the incidence of melanoma and prostate cancer.[43,44] This and other findings suggest that immune genetic markers can predict cancer growth. At present, however, it remains unknown whether genetic factors associated with immune function can modulate response to therapy either in the context of systemic administration of immune modulators such as IL-2 or IFNα or in the context of antigen-specific immunization. Future work should address genetic polymorphism associated with distinct immunologically related genes since techniques suitable for the screening of polymorphisms in clinical settings at a genome-wide level are currently becoming available.[1,45]

It is, however, likely that the heterogeneity of tumors may play a key role in determining immune responsiveness. This impression is based on the relatively common, though poorly documented in the literature observation of the mixed responses. Melanoma and renal cell cancer are the most sensitive cancers to immunotherapy. These cancers have a propensity to spontaneous partial regressions that affect often individual metastases while others simultaneously grow. This phenomenon is often enhanced by therapy. Multiple lesions in patients with metastatic melanoma or renal cell cancer may respond differently to immunotherapy; some may regress while others simultaneously progress in response to the same treatment. Considering the genetic background and immune status of the individual bearing such lesions as a constant, the observation of the mixed responses suggests that different conditions in the tumor micro-environments may strongly affect the outcome of anticancer immune responses.

Gene Profiling of Anticancer Immune Responses

Gene profiling provides investigators with new opportunities, particularly in circumstances when too little is known about biological events such as those regulating tumor/host interactions that are too complex to allow the formulation of plausible hypotheses.[46] We provided some examples of how gene profiling could provide pattern recognition tools that could be used for identification of characteristics specific of lesions likely to respond to immunotherapy. FNA were obtained from subcutaneous melanoma metastases prior to immunotherapy leaving the lesions in place.[38] This strategy allowed the direct linking of biological information with the clinical outcome. Previous gene profiling studies suggested that melanomas segregate into two molecular subclasses representing distinct taxonomies.[47] These observations were based on the profiling of cell lines or tissue preparations which were not linked to clinical information regarding outcome of therapy and overall survival. The subsequent prospective collection of clinical information and biological samples with FNA allowed direct correlation of the gene expression profile to clinical parameters. In addition, as serial FNA samples of the same lesions could be collected, it was possible to monitor the changes in the transcriptional profile occurring with time and/or in response to therapy in individual lesions adding, therefore, a temporal dimension to the study of cancer biology. This strategy demonstrated that the two melanoma subclasses did not represent two distinct disease taxonomies but rather two stages of the same genetically unstable disease rapidly evolving in natural conditions and/or in response to therapy.[48] In addition it was also possible to directly link genetic profiling with clinical history. By separating lesions that responded from those that did not respond to active specific immunization combined with systemic IL-2 administration, we could identify genes predictive of immune responsiveness. The genetic profile characteristic of immune responsiveness was remarkable, particularly because most of the genes included were associated with immune function. This suggests that tumor deposits likely to respond to immune therapy are preconditioned to response by a tumor micro-environment immunologically active even before treatment administration.[38] In particular, the identification of IFN-regulatory factor-2 (IRF-2) over-expression in lesions likely to respond suggested that immune responsive tumors are chronically inflamed before treatment. This inflammatory process may not be sufficient to induce tumor rejection but it may favor the induction of acute inflammation during therapy by recruiting immune cells at the tumor site.[49] A paired analysis of FNA samples obtained before and during therapy supported this possibility, as lesions that underwent complete response over-expressed IRF-1, which is a marker of acute inflammation.[50] Thus, this pattern recognition analysis suggested that immune responsiveness is predetermined by the presence of a chronic inflammatory status reminiscent of chronic, therapy controlled allograft rejection that can be turned into acute inflammation by immune manipulation as acute allograft rejection may overcome immune suppression under environmentally-induced immune stimulation. Some have suggested that inflammation is beneficial and necessary for tumor growth.[51,52] Our observations are only apparently contrasting with this hypothesis since inflammation may promote angiogenesis and cell growth through the release of growth and angio-regulatory factors during tissue remodeling and repair. Similarly, growth factors produced by tumor cells may enhance their effect through an autocrine mechanism of self stimulation or they may mimic the normal repair-promoting response of the organism to injury stimulating angiogenesis and recruitment of stroma formation-promoting cells which may benefit tumor growth. However, the same growth factors may act on immune cells since several of them have chemo-attractant and regulatory properties on immune cells. These molecules can induce the migration of cells of the innate and adaptive immune system within the tumor micro-environment. Such cells alone are probably not able to exert anticancer properties, but could rapidly turn into powerful effector anticancer cells given appropriate stimulatory conditions, which may be induced by treatment such as the systemic administration of IL-2.[53] Thus, pattern recognition allowed the formulation of a novel hypothesis about the mechanism of immune response.

Gene profiling of melanoma metastases identified a large number of genes over-expressed in the micro-environment of melanoma metastases that code for lymphokines, cytokines, growth factors and metalloproteases. Interestingly, the expression of most of these genes is coordinate among different tumors.[3] In particular, we noted that the expression of most cytokines and growth factors was tightly associated with the over-expression of genes related to the function of interferons, suggesting that the presence of molecules with pro-inflammatory function is associated with correspondent intracellular signaling, probably downstream of their ligand interaction. These finding support the previous statement that in some tumors cancer cells evolve to produce a wealth of pro-inflammatory, growth promoting, angio-regulatory immune-reactive molecules that can simultaneously foster tumor growth through autocrine or paracrine paths while recruiting immune effector mechanisms that may, in appropriate conditions, turn against their own growth.

Systemic IL-2 administration seems on occasions to facilitate the switch from chronic to acute inflammation required for tumor regression. This cytokine is a powerful anticancer agent which acts indirectly through immune activation. Although clinical responses are relatively rare, their dramatic occurrence is characterized by a rapid disappearance of large tumor bulks and, in some instances, long-term disease-free survival.[32] Independently from its therapeutic value, the effects of IL-2 are of extreme biological interest. IL-2 is believed to act in favor of immune-mediated cancer regression by facilitating the passage of tumor-specific T-cells from the circulation to the tumor site through an increase in blood vessel permeability.[54] It is also believed that IL-2 acts in vivo as a growth factor or activator of CD8$^+$ T-cells[55] or through the activation of intra-tumoral endothelial cells, which may in turn promote migration of TA-specific T-cells within tumors.[56] It is also likely that IL-2 may act through the secondary production of an extensive array of cytokines by primary stimulation of circulating mononuclear cells. The subsequent cytokine storm may have broad immune/pro-inflammatory effects and may provide the costimulation necessary for the full activation of TA-specific T-cells and other immune effector cells.[53,57] The analysis of early transcriptional changes in circulating mononuclear cells exposed to IL-2 administration identified similarities with those occurring within the tumor micro-environment of melanoma metastases. Serial FNA of melanoma metastases performed before and during systemic IL-2 administration suggested that the immediate effect of systemic IL-2 administration on peripheral mononuclear cells and more dramatically in the tumor micro-environment is a transcriptional activation of genes predominantly associated with monocyte function, while minimal effects occur on migration, activation and proliferation of T-cells.[53] Thus, IL-2 induces inflammation at tumor sites by activating antigen-presenting monocytes, inducing a broad production of chemo-attractants and activating innate cytotoxic mechanisms in monocytes and natural killer cells which in turn contribute to the induction of an acute inflammatory condition necessary for T cell recruitment, activation and proliferation.

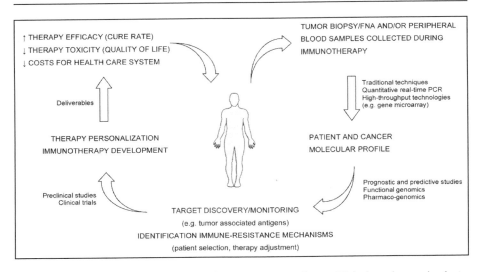

Figure 1. A scheme of the translational approach to cancer immunotherapy. High-throughput technologies such as gene micorarray can speed up the process of data collection from cancer patients undergoing immunotherapy. This information is believed to be essential to dissect the reasons of immunotherapy failure and thus to improve currently available immunotherapeutic strategies.

Conclusions

The previous examples illustrate how high throughput tools can be applied to study of complex biological processes in their entirety such as those regulating tumor/host interactions.[16] The study of individual genetic predisposition to disease and response to treatment[1,45] could be combined with that of epigenetic changes during life and disease progression[16] and that of real-time adaptation of the transcriptional profile of biological samples in relevant conditions.[16] The most significant problem remains the availability of relevant samples of a quality worth studying. Thus, carefully and prospectively collected samples should be obtained during the conduct of clinical trials in the future to understand the biology of cancer cells, their relationship with the host and their response/adaptation to therapy.[11] Only the extensive application of such translational medicine approach will provide investigators with the scientific information needed to improve immunotherapy protocols in order to obtain clinically valuable and durable control of cancer (Fig. 1).

References

1. Jin P, Wang E. Polymorphism in clinical immunology - From HLA typing to immunogenetic profiling. J Transl Med 2003; 1(1):8.
2. Marincola FM, Jaffee EM, Hicklin DJ et al. Escape of human solid tumors from T-cell recognition: Molecular mechanisms and functional significance. Adv Immunol 2000; 74:181-273.
3. Marincola FM, Wang E, Herlyn M et al. Tumors as elusive targets of T-cell-based active immunotherapy. Trends Immunol 2003; 24(6):335-342.
4. Wang E, Marincola FM. cDNA arrays and the enigma of melanoma immune responsiveness. Cancer J 2001; 7(1):16-24.
5. Dunn GP, Bruce AT, Ikeda H et al. Cancer immunoediting: From immunosurveillance to tumor escape. Nat Immunol 2002; 3(11):991-998.
6. Aichele P, Brduscha-Riem K, Oehen S et al. Peptide antigen treatment of naive and virus-immune mice: Antigen-specific tolerance versus immunopathology. Immunity 1997; 6(5):519-529.
7. Zinkernagel RM. Immunology taught by viruses. Science 1996; 271(5246):173-178.
8. Ochsenbein AF, Klenerman P, Karrer U et al. Immune surveillance against a solid tumor fails because of immunological ignorance. Proc Natl Acad Sci USA 1999; 96(5):2233-2238.

9. Fuchs EJ, Matzinger P. Is cancer dangerous to the immune system? Semin Immunol 1996; 8(5):271-280.
10. Matzinger P. Introduction to the series. Danger model of immunity. Scand J Immunol 2001; 54(1-2):2-3.
11. Marincola FM. Translational medicine: A two-way road. J Transl Med 2003; 1(1):1.
12. Yang JC, Rosenberg SA. An ongoing prospective randomized comparison of interleukin-2 regimens for the treatment of metastatic renal cell cancer. Cancer J Sci Am 1997; 3(Suppl 1):S79-S84.
13. Schwab ED, Pienta KJ. Cancer as a complex adaptive system. Med Hypotheses 1996; 47(3):235-241.
14. Cucuianu A. Chaos in cancer? Nat Med 1998; 4(12):1342-1343.
15. Dalgleish A. The relevance of nonlinear mathematics (chaos theory) to the treatment of cancer, the role of the immune response and the potential for vaccines. Q J Med 1999; 92(6):347-359.
16. Wang E, Panelli MC, Marincola FM. Genomic analysis of cancer. Princ Pract Oncol 2003; 17(9):1-16.
17. Wang E, Marincola FM. A natural history of melanoma: Serial gene expression analysis. Immunol Today 2000; 21(12):619-623.
18. Monsurro V, Wang E, Panelli MC et al. Active-specific immunization against melanoma: Is the problem at the receiving end? Semin Cancer Biol 2003; 13(6):473-480.
19. Andersen MH, Gehl J, Reker S et al. Dynamic changes of specific T cell responses to melanoma correlate with IL-2 administration. Semin Cancer Biol 2003; 13(6):449-459.
20. Parmiani G, Castelli C, Rivoltini L et al. Immunotherapy of melanoma. Semin Cancer Biol 2003; 13(6):391-400.
21. Horig H, Kaufman HL. Local delivery of poxvirus vaccines for melanoma. Semin Cancer Biol 2003; 13(6):417-422.
22. Scheibenbogen C, Letsch A, Schmittel A et al. Rational peptide-based tumor vaccine development and T cell monitoring. Semin Cancer Biol 2003; 13(6):423-429.
23. Talebi T, Weber JS. Peptide vaccine trials for melanoma: Preclinical background and clinical results. Semin Cancer Biol 2003; 13(6):431-438.
24. Paczesny S, Ueno H, Fay J et al. Dendritic cells as vectors for immunotherapy of cancer. Semin Cancer Biol 2003; 13(6):439-447.
25. Speiser DE, Pittet MJ, Rimoldi D et al. Evaluation of melanoma vaccines with molecularly defined antigens by ex vivo monitoring of tumor specific T cells. Semin Cancer Biol 2003; 13(6):461-472.
26. Kaech SM, Hemby S, Kersh E et al. Molecular and functional profiling of memory CD8 T cell differentiation. Cell 2002; 111(6):837-851.
27. Wherry EJ, Teichgraber V, Becker TC et al. Lineage relationship and protective immunity of memory CD8 T cell subsets. Nat Immunol 2003; 4(3):225-234.
28. Monsurro V, Nagorsen D, Wang E et al. Functional heterogeneity of vaccine-induced CD8+ T cells. J Immunol 2002; 168(11):5933-5942.
29. Monsurro V, Wang E, Yamano Y et al. Quiescent phenotype of tumor-specific CD8+ T cells following immunization. Blood 2004; 104(7):1970-8.
30. Wang E, Miller LD, Ohnmacht GA et al. High-fidelity mRNA amplification for gene profiling. Nat Biotechnol 2000; 18(4):457-459.
31. Wang E, Marincola FM. Amplification of small quantities of mRNA for transcript analysis. In: Bowtell D, Sambrook J, eds. DNA Arrays - A Molecular Cloning Manual. NY, USA: Cold Spring Harbor Laboratory Press, 2002:204-213.
32. Atkins MB, Lotze MT, Dutcher JP et al. High-dose recombinant interleukin-2 therapy for patients with metastatic melanoma: Analysis of 270 patients treated between 1985 and 1993. J Clin Oncol 1998; 17(7):2105-2116.
33. Kammula US, Lee K-H, Riker AI et al. Functional analysis of antigen-specific T lymphocytes by serial measurement of gene expression in peripheral blood mononuclear cells and tumor specimens. J Immunol 1999; 163(12):6867-6875.
34. Wolfel T, Klehmann E, Muller C et al. Lysis of human melanoma cells by autologous cytolytic T cell clones. Identification of human histocompatibility leukocyte antigen A2 as a restriction element for three different antigens. J Exp Med 1989; 170(3):797-810.
35. Panelli MC, Riker A, Kammula U et al. Expansion of tumor-T cell pairs from fine needle aspirates of melanoma metastases. J Immunol 2000; 164(1):495-504.
36. Pockaj BA, Sherry RM, Wei JP et al. Localization of [111]indium-labeled tumor infiltrating lymphocytes to tumor in patients receiving adoptive immunotherapy. Augmentation with cyclophosphamide and correlation with response. Cancer 1994; 73(6):1731-1737.
37. Ohnmacht GA, Wang E, Mocellin S et al. Short-term kinetics of tumor antigen expression in response to vaccination. J Immunol 2001; 167(3):1809-1820.

38. Wang E, Miller LD, Ohnmacht GA et al. Prospective molecular profiling of melanoma metastases suggests classifiers of immune responsiveness. Cancer Res 2002; 62(13):3581-3586.

39. Wang E, Marincola FM, Stroncek D. Human leukocyte antigen (HLA) and human neutrophil antigen (HNA) systems. In: Hoffman R, Benz EJ, Shattil SJ et al, eds. Hematology: Basic Principles and Practice. PA, USA: Elsevier Science, 2003.

40. Rubin JT, Adams SD, Simonis T et al. HLA polymorphism and response to IL-2 bases therapy in patients with melanoma. Proc Soc Biol Ther Annu Meet 1991; 1:18.

41. Marincola FM, Shamamian P, Rivoltini L et al. HLA associations in the antitumor response against malignant melanoma. J Immunother Emphasis Tumor Immunol 1995; 18(4):242-252.

42. Lee JE, Reveille JD, Ross MI et al. HLA-DQB1*0301 association with increased cutaneous melanoma risk. Int J Cancer 1994; 59(4):510-513.

43. Howell WM, Bateman AC, Turner SJ et al. Influence of vascular endothelial growth factor single nucleotide polymorphisms on tumour development in cutaneous malignant melanoma. Genes Immun 2002; 3(4):229-232.

44. Howell WM, Calder PC, Grimble RF. Gene polymorphisms, inflammatory diseases and cancer. Proc Nutr Soc 2002; 61(4):447-456.

45. Wang E, Adams S, Zhao Y et al. A strategy for detection of known and unknown SNP using a minimum number of oligonucleotides applicable in the clinical settings. J Transl Med 2003; 1(1):4.

46. Marincola FM. Mechanisms of immune escape and immune tolerance. In: Rosenberg SA, ed. Principles and Practice of the Biologic Therapy of Cancer. Philadelphia, USA: Lippincott Williams and Wilkins, 2000:601-617.

47. Bittner M, Meltzer P, Chen Y et al. Molecular classification of cutaneous malignant melanoma by gene expression profiling. Nature 2000; 406(6795):536-540.

48. Lengauer C, Kinzler KW, Vogelstein B. Genetic instabilities in human cancers. Nature 1998; 396(6712):643-649.

49. Mocellin S, Panelli MC, Wang E et al. The dual role of IL-10. Trends Immunol 2003; 24(1):36-43.

50. Taniguchi T. Transcription factors IRF-1 and IRF-2: Linking the immune responses and tumor suppression. J Cell Physiol 1997; 173(2):128-130.

51. Daniel D, Meyer-Morse N, Bergsland EK et al. Immune enhancement of skin carcinogenesis by CD4+ T cells. J Exp Med 2003; 197(8):1017-1028.

52. Hanahan D, Lanzavecchia A, Mihich E. Fourteenth Annual Pezcoller Symposium: The novel dichotomy of immune interactions with tumors. Cancer Res 2003; 63(11):3005-3008.

53. Panelli MC, Wang E, Phan G et al. Gene-expression profiling of the response of peripheral mononuclear cells and melanoma metastases in response to systemic IL-2 administration. Genome Biol 2002; 3(7):RESEARCH0035.

54. Rosenberg SA, Yang JC, Schwartzentruber DJ et al. Immunologic and therapeutic evaluation of a synthetic peptide vaccine for the treatment of patients with metastatic melanoma. Nat Med 1998; 4(3):321-327.

55. Margolin KA. Interleukin-2 in the treatment of renal cancer. Semin Oncol 2000; 27(2):194-203.

56. Cotran RS, Pober JS, Gimbrone Jr MA et al. Endothelial activation during interleukin 2 immunotherapy. A possible mechanism for the vascular leak syndrome. J Immunol 1988; 140(6):1883-1888.

57. Kasid A, Director EP, Rosenberg SA. Induction of endogenous cytokine-mRNA in circulating peripheral blood mononuclear cells by IL-2 administration to cancer patients. J Immunol 1989; 143(2):736-739.

CHAPTER 8

Identification of Molecular Determinants of Tumor Sensitivity and Resistance to Anticancer Drugs

Luigi Quintieri,* Marianna Fantin and Csaba Vizler

Abstract

Resistance to drugs is a major problem in cancer chemotherapy. Various cellular mechanisms of drug resistance have been identified in cultured tumor cell lines selected for growth in the presence of sublethal concentrations of various anticancer drugs. They involve drug transport and detoxification, qualitative or quantitative alterations of the drug target, repair of drug-induced DNA lesions, and alterations in signaling or execution of apoptosis. More recently, the possibility to simultaneously analyze the expression of thousands of genes using DNA microarrays has allowed exploring the relationships between gene expression and sensitivity to several anticancer drugs. A number of studies using microarrays for identifying genes governing tumor chemosensitivity focused on tumor cell lines. Some clinical studies have also been carried out to investigate whether tumor gene expression patterns could predict clinical response to chemotherapy. Results of these studies are encouraging, indicating that individualization of drug treatment based on multigenic response-predictive markers is feasible.

Introduction

Given alone or in combination, chemotherapeutic drugs produce a significant clinical impact on various cancers such as germ cell, small cell lung and bladder carcinomas where overall response rates can exceed 90%.[1] Furthermore, in many common cancer (e.g., non small cell lung, colorectal and ovarian cancer) substantial tumor shrinkage can be expected in more than 50% of cases. However, in other cases, response rates are lower; e.g., only 10-20% of patients with melanoma, renal cell, pancreatic and esophageal carcinomas respond to current available drug therapy.

Clinically speaking, tumor resistance to chemotherapy can either be intrinsic or acquired. Intrinsic resistance is present at the time of diagnosis in tumors that fail to respond to first-line chemotherapy. Acquired resistance occurs in tumors that are initially highly responsive to therapy, but on relapse exhibit a different phenotype being resistant to both previously used drugs and, frequently, also to new agents with a different chemical structure and mode of action.

The major known causes of tumor resistance to drugs fall into two groups; firstly, those leading to impaired delivery of drugs to target cells or altering how a tumor cell responds to

*Corresponding Author: Luigi Quintieri—Pharmacology Section, Department of Pharmacology and Anesthesiology, University of Padova, Largo Meneghetti, 2, I-35131 Padova, Italy. Email: luigi.quintieri@unipd.it

Microarray Technology and Cancer Gene Profiling, edited by Simone Mocellin.
©2007 Landes Bioscience and Springer Science+Business Media.

cytotoxic drugs (e.g., cell adhesion-mediated drug resistance; see below); secondly, genetic alterations in the cancer cell itself affecting cell sensitivity to drugs (referred below as "tumor cell-specific mechanisms of drug resistance"). Insufficient drug delivery to target cells can result from poor absorption of orally administered drugs, increased metabolic inactivation by host enzymes and/or increased excretion, resulting in lower levels of drug in the blood and in decreased diffusion of drugs from the blood to the tumor mass.[2,3] Furthermore, recent studies have stressed the role of heterogeneous tumor blood supply in limiting uniform drug delivery to the target tissue.[3] A further determinant of response to anticancer drugs is the tumoral microenvironment. Experimental models demonstrate that when tumor cells have established contact with their environment, i.e., extracellular matrix components, stromal cells, endothelial cells or tumor cells in a three-dimensional system, they become less sensitive to anticancer drugs. In particular, interaction of tumor cell adhesion molecules (e.g., β_1 integrins) with various extracellular matrix proteins (e.g., fibronectin, laminin and collagen IV) can contributes to drug resistance in vivo via suppression of chemotherapy-induced apoptosis;[4,5] this form of drug resistance has been given the term "cell adhesion-mediated drug resistance". Moreover, secretion of anti-apoptotic growth factors by tumor-associated stromal cells seems to play a role in the drug resistance of certain types of tumors such as multiple myeloma and pancreatic carcinoma.[6,7]

Different types of tumor cell-specific mechanisms of drug resistance have been identified, mainly by exposing tumor cell lines in culture to increasing concentrations of anticancer drugs and analyzing the surviving clones for chromosomal alterations, gene and/or protein expression and phenotype. These include: (a) overexpression of ATP-dependent efflux pumps, e.g., those belonging to the family of ATP-binding cassette transporters such as P-glycoprotein and multidrug-resistance-associated protein 1, that prevent drugs, such as classical anthracyclines and paclitaxel (Taxol™), to reach their intracellular targets;[8] (b) increased intratumoral detoxification of the drug and/or its active metabolite(s) by enzymes such as the glutathione-S-transferases;[9] (c) quantitative or qualitative alterations of the drug's cellular targets, e.g., mutations in *β-tubulin* and *Bcr-Abl* genes conferring resistance to paclitaxel and imatinib (Gleevec™), respectively;[10-12] (e) quantitative or qualitative alterations in genes coding for proteins involved in apoptotic pathways such as inactivating mutations of *p53* and overexpression of anti-apoptotic proteins (e.g., BCL-2);[13] and (f) deregulation of DNA repair mechanisms, such as deficiency of mismatch repair, causing drug resistance (evasion of drug-induced apoptosis) through the failure of tumor cells to recognize DNA damage.[14] Finally, it is well known that the cytotoxicity of several antitumor agents, the so-called cell cycle-specific drugs, rely on the position of the cells in the cell cycle; this explain why, in combination therapy approaches, administration of one anticancer drug leading to arrest in a specific phase of the cell cycle can reduce the effectiveness of the next drug given immediately in sequence and having maximum toxicity in a different phase of the cell cycle.[15]

An important principle in anticancer drug resistance is that tumor cell populations within tumor masses are fundamentally heterogeneous, as the genetic instability of tumor cells results in the emergence of subpopulations harboring various genetic alterations, and differing in a wide range of cellular characteristics, including sensitivity to anticancer drugs.[16] So, in any population of tumor cells that is exposed to chemotherapy, more than one mechanism of cellular drug resistance can be active. This explains why modulation of a single drug-resistance marker, such as P-glycoprotein overexpression, has proven to be of limited benefit in the clinic.[17]

Because there are presently no proven predictors of a patient's response to chemotherapy, all cancer patients selected for chemotherapy receive the same treatment. The availability of tools for prediction of cancer sensitivity to chemotherapy would be of high value for the management of individual patients allowing the clinical oncologist to choose the single agent or the drug combination the most likely to elicit a positive response while keeping host toxicity under acceptable levels.

Correlation of Gene Expression Data from DNA Arrays with Response to Anticancer Agents

The DNA Microarray Technology

The gene expression profile of a cell determines its phenotype and its response to various factors, including drugs. Up until the recent past, researchers were only able to examine the expression levels of one or a few genes at a time but with the advent of microarray technology, more than 30,000 genes can be analyzed at once. Obviously, this technology is transforming how biomedical research is carried out, allowing for a more complete analysis of complex diseases such as cancer. In brief, a DNA microarray consists of a solid support (a glass, nylon, plastic or nitrocellulose slide) coated with many spots, each of which contains many immobilized identical single-stranded complementary DNA (cDNA) sequences or oligonucleotides (often called "probes") representing a target gene. To analyze gene expression with DNA microarrays, RNA is extracted from tissue or cells and, most commonly, subjected to simultaneous reverse transcription and fluorescence or radioactive labeling. This procedure led to the obtaining of a sample mixture containing many different sequences of labeled cDNA in various amounts, corresponding to the numbers of copies of the original messenger RNA (mRNA) species extracted from the sample. The mixture is then added to the microarray slide; through the base pairing principle described by Watson and Crick, the labeled cDNA binds to the DNA sequences immobilized on the slide (hybridization). After washes and image acquisition, the signal of each spot is automatically detected and quantified with specialized software; it is proportional to the concentration of the corresponding mRNA species in the original tissue or cell sample, in other words, to the expression level of the considered gene. Intensities are then normalized and converted into expression levels, absolute or relative depending on the approach, and these are analyzed with bioinformatic tools and stored in databases.

Basal Gene Expression Profiling of Tumor Cell Lines and Response to Anticancer Drugs

Beyond using DNA microarrays for diagnostic and prognostic purposes, researchers also employ this technology to identify genes involved in drug sensitivity or resistance to anticancer drugs. One strategy is to establish basal gene expression profiles for a panel of tumor cell lines, and also to measure cytotoxic activity (or another cellular parameter) for a list of antitumor agents in the same tumor cell panel. It is then possible to attempt to correlate the activity of each agent to the gene expression profile of each tumor cell line. The first example of this type of study is that performed by Scherf and collegues[18] using a cDNA microarray. These researchers analyzed the gene expression patterns of a panel of 60 untreated human tumor cell lines (termed "NCI60") used by the Developmental Therapeutic Program (DTP) of the United States National Cancer Institute (NCI) to screen >100,000 compounds since 1990. The gene expression data (available at http://discover.nci.nih.gov) were then analyzed for correlation with the growth inhibitory activity of a subset of ~70,000 compounds previously tested in the same tumor cell lines [these growth inhibition data can be found at the NCI DTP website (http://dtp.nci.nih.gov)]. The study focused on 1,376 genes (out of a total of 9,703 gene transcripts) that showed the larger variations across the cell lines, and the activity of 118 drugs with known mechanisms of action. Correlation analysis revealed many highly significant drug activity - gene expression relationships. Whereas some of them were expected, such as that linking the expression of dihydropyrimidine dehydrogenase and resistance to 5-fluorouracil (5-FU), which is consistent with the notion that dihydropyrimidine dehydrogenase is involved in the cellular catabolism of 5-FU, most of them remain to be understood and investigated. Since the pioneering work done at NCI by Scherf and collegues[18] the techniques of evaluation of gene expression profiles have evolved, and the number of gene probes available has increased; however this work represents a cornerstone for DNA microarray-based studies on genes governing sensitivity/resistance to anticancer drugs. Moreover, the availability of these data on public websites allows everybody to perform data exploration.

Several studies have pursued and extended the work of NCI using the NCI60 cancer cell line cytotoxicity database and either the original gene expression profile database established at Stanford[18] or those established by Millenium Corporation (also available on the DTP website) and by the Whitehead Institute for Biomedical Research (see below; http://www.broad.mit.edu/cancer) using oligonucleotide microarrays (Affymetrix technology). Among them, the study carried out by Staunton and colleagues at the Whitehead Institute, aimed at the development of classifiers, i.e., gene clusters capable of predicting sensitivity or resistance to 232 drugs in the NCI60 cell panel.[19] In general, the classifiers were complex and difficult to interpret. However this analysis identified some understandable drug - target relationships. For example, the classifier for cytochalasin D, a cytotoxic compound which binds to actin and interferes with its polymerization, included 29 genes (out of a total of 120) related to cytoskeleton or extracellular matrix. This suggested that these types of studies could reveal information on factors governing drug resistance/sensitivity, in addition to providing information on the potential target.

The work of Masumarra and collegues[20] examined the original NCI60 gene expression and cytotoxicity screening databases using a powerful multivariate statistical procedure, called "partial least squares modelling in latent variables or projections to latent structures", and identified the relationships between the cytotoxicity of 171 drugs with known and unknown mechanism action and expression of 9,605 transcripts. Six gene products appeared to influence response to topoisomerase II inhibitors, RNA/DNA antimetabolites and alkylating agents (i.e., response to DNA damaging agents), but not to the antimitotics. Not surprisingly, some of the genes found to influence response to antimitotics affects the structure of cytoskeleton.

A study by Blower and colleagues[21] describes the use of a "structure-activity-target" statistical approach to identify molecular structural features that are found in compounds whose activity patterns are highly correlated with expression patterns of selected genes in the NCI60 cell panel. Sensitivity to two classes of compounds, benzothiophenediones and indolonaphtoquinones was found to be correlated (positively or negatively) with several genes in melanoma and leukaemia cell lines. In particular, while the activity of benzothiophenediones bearing electron-donating substituents was positively correlated to the expression of several genes over-expressed in melanoma cell lines, the cytotoxicity of members of the same family having electron-withdrawing substituents was not or negatively correlated with those genes. This study suggests that the "structure-activity-target" approach can be used to prioritize candidate compounds for more detailed drug-gene correlation analysis or further biological studies and thus has the potential to accelerate the process of drug discovery.

More recently, a further in silico research has been conducted mining the freely available databases of the NCI in an attempt to identify the molecular determinants of the activity of four platinum compounds, namely, cisplatin, carboplatin, oxaliplatin and tetraplatin.[22] Some genes whose expression was found to be correlated to the cytotoxic activity of platinum compounds were already known as determinants of drug activity: this is the case of *ERB*-B2 and *BCL*-X_L genes, whose expression correlated negatively with the cytotoxicity of all four compounds. Interestingly, the activity of oxaliplatin and tetraplatin was significantly higher in cell lines with an overexpression of the *c-MYC* gene, whereas there was no correlation between *c-MYC* expression and the activity of cisplatin and carboplatin. This may suggest that patients bearing tumors overexpressing this gene could be particularly responsive to oxaliplatin.

Another study by Huang and collegues[23] used oligonucleotide arrays to analyze expression of genes coding for ion channels and membrane transporters in the NCI60 cell panel. Gene expression data were then analyzed for correlation with the growth inhibition data of 119 drugs which had been previously obtained by the DTP program (http://dtp.nci.nih.gov). The analysis revealed several significant gene-drug correlation, many of which corresponded to known transporter-drug substrate relationships, thus validating the approach and suggesting a prominent role for membrane transporter in determining chemosensitivity. For example, expression of genes coding for folate, nucleoside, and amino acid transporters positively correlated with sensitivity to their respective drug substrates. Moreover, three ATP-binding cassette genes (MDR1, *ABCC3,* and *ABCC5*) showed significant negative correlations with the sensitivity to several cytotoxic drugs.

Few academic or industrial structures can afford the development of large databases such as those above-mentioned. The Japanese Foundation for Cancer Research has published in 2002 two studies inspired from the NCI approach. The first study used microarrays to determine the expression pattern of 9,216 genes in a panel of 39 human tumor cell lines (termed "JFCR-39") and integrated the data with the in vitro cytotoxicity profile of 55 anticancer agents.[24] This study identified some genes, e.g., *aldose reductase* and *damage-specific DNA binding protein 2,* showing positive correlation with sensitivity to various drugs, indicating that they could be common markers of chemosensitivity. Moreover other genes, such as *LIM domain protein kinase 2,* involved in actin skeleton remodeling, exhibited a negative correlation with responsiveness to several drugs, and might therefore represent common markers of drug resistance; correlations were also observed with specific classes of drugs. For example, expression levels of *survivin* and *apoptosis inhibitor 1,* both involved in apoptosis, were negatively correlated with sensitivity to 5-FU derivatives. The second study used a cDNA microarray representing 23,040 genes to analyze expression profiles in a panel of 85 human tumors xenografted in nude mice.[25] Furthermore, the xenografts were examined for sensitivity to nine commonly used anticancer agents. Correlation analysis found certain associations between gene expression and sensitivity to the tested anticancer agents that were interesting; for example a negative correlation was found between *thymidilate synthetase* expression and 5-FU, and also a negative correlation was observed between *aldehyde dehydrogenase 1* and sensitivity to camptothecin.

A third study from the same institution, published in 2005,[26] established a new panel of 45 human tumor cell lines (named "JFCR-45") derived from tumors arising from three different organs, i.e., breast, liver and stomach. All cell lines were analyzed for sensitivity to 53 anticancer drugs, allowing the development a database of chemosensitivity. Forty-two cell lines of JFCR-45 were also examined for gene expression using a cDNA array consisting of 3,537 genes. Correlation analysis between chemosensitivity and gene expression profiles identified many genes correlated with respect to the sensitivity of each drug. Among these, *JUN* and *heat shock protein 1A1* (*HSPA1A*) were positively correlated with sensitivity to mitomycin C.

Another research group evaluated the sensitivity to eight anticancer drugs and gene expression profiles in eight human hepatoma cell lines, and then analyzed the data by constructing relevance networks.[27] The study identified 42 genes that showed significant correlation to drug responsiveness; almost 20% of these code for membrane transporter proteins, most of which were negatively correlated with chemosensitivity. For example, expression of *transporter associated with antigen processing-1* (*TAP1*) was negatively correlated with sensitivity to mitoxantrone. In addition, a negative correlation was observed between expression of *topoisomerase II\beta* and sensitivity to doxorubicin, and also a negative correlation was identified between *aldehyde dehydrogenase 1* and sensitivity to camptothecin.

Mariadason and colleagues[28] established a panel of 30 colorectal carcinoma cell lines, and evaluated both the constitutive gene expression profiles and their sensitivity to 5-FU- and camptothecin-induced apoptosis. They identified groups of 50 and 149 genes whose expression was highly predictive of 5-FU and camptothecin-induced apoptosis respectively. Moreover, they demonstrated that gene expression profiling approach predicted response more effectively than the four previously established determinants of 5-FU response: i.e., thymidylate synthase and thymidine phosphorylase activity, and p53 and mismatch repair status.

Critical Comments on Tumor Cell Line Gene Expression Profile-Drug Sensitivity Correlation Studies

The approaches described above sound very promising. However there are several potential drawback that can be addressed.

1. The cell lines have been selected for growth in culture and may not reflect the phenotype of the tumor from which they were isolated from. In particular, as discussed above, in vivo interactions between the stroma and tumor are probably critical parameters in chemosensitivity.

2. The DNA microarray techniques are still imperfect and this may be the source of discrepancies that are observed between studies. A critical analysis has examined three gene expression databases corresponding to the NCI60 human tumor cell line panel (i.e., the Stanford, the Millenium and the Whitehead datasets), and the relationship of these to the corresponding growth inhibition data.[29] Among the 2,105 genes common to the three databases (representing less than 10% of the human genome) only 11 were found to be correlated in all studies, indicating absence of reproducibility. Moreover, although DNA arrays contain thousands of genes, their limited sensitivity and precision restrict the analysis to those genes whose expression shows sufficiently large variations in expression across the samples analyzed.

3. For reasons of automation and reproducibility, the drug activity databases have been frequently generated from a single end-point of growth delay at 48 h, which is a measure of short-term growth inhibition and/or cytotoxic activity. Since in vivo tumor response is determined by tumor cell kill,[30] and there is no reason to suppose that drug-induced short-term growth inhibition should correlate with drug-induced cell kill, the gene-drug sensitivity correlations observed in these studies may not be relevant in the clinical situation.

4. Conclusion drawn from these approaches rely on the establishment of a correlation. However the relationship between drug activity and gene expression do not always indicate causal relationship. For example if expression of the gene A is linearly correlated with that of the gene B, both genes may show a correlation with the same drug, but only one has a real causal link.

Profiling Gene Expression Changes in Response to Drug Treatment

All of the studies discussed above were based on the gene expression profiling of wild-type (drug-untreated) tumor cells. However, several in vitro studies focused on the gene expression alterations occurring in tumor cells in response to anticancer drugs or have addressed differential gene expression patterns between drug-sensitive cell lines and those with acquired resistance.

Kudoh and collegues[31] evaluated the gene expression profile of MCF-7 breast cancer cells that were either transiently treated with doxorubicin or selected for resistance to the same drug (MCF-7/D40). Several genes, such as *26S proteasome regulatory subunit 4*, and *epoxide hydrolase*, have been found to be constitutively overexpressed in MCF-7/D40 doxorubicin-resistant cells. These genes were also induced by doxorubicin treatment of MCF-7 wild-type cells but were not found in MCF-7 cisplatin-resistant cells. Based on these findings the authors suggested that these genes may represent a signature profile of resistance to doxorubicin. The approach adopted by the authors is intriguing because the candidate resistance genes are cross-validated through two distinct approaches.

A similar study[32] used a 5,760-gene cDNA microarray with the aim to identify genes involved in the multidrug-resistance phenotype. The researchers compared the gene expression profile of the parental multiple myeloma cell line RPMI 8226 with that of its doxorubicin-selected sublines 8226/Dox6 and 8226/Dox40, both of which express P-glycoprotein and are multidrug-resistant. The microarray analysis detected the differential expression of 380 genes, many of which having a role in apoptotic signaling, and probably contributing to the multidrug-resistance phenotype.

Zhou and coworkers[33] evaluated the transcriptional response of HCT116 human colon cancer cells, upon synchronization in the S phase of the cell cycle, to two different concentrations of the topoisomerase I inhibitor camptothecin. Short-term incubation with 20 and 1,000 nM camptothecin caused reversible and irreversible G2 arrest, respectively, and the patterns of gene expression change (with reference to untreated controls) were noticeably different at the two concentrations. In particular, a group of genes, including known DNA damage-inducible genes and also genes associated with cell cycle arrest and apoptosis (e.g., the cyclin-dependent kinase inhibitor *p21* and the apoptosis-inducer *CD95/Fas*) were upregulated only in response to the higher concentration of the drug. Based on these findings, the authors proposed that there is a fundamental difference between the gene expression changes associated with reversible G2 delay that follows mild DNA damage and permanent G2 arrest that follows more extensive DNA damage.

Reinhold and colleagues[34] used cDNA arrays to compare the gene expression profile of a DU145-derived human prostate cancer line selected for resistance to the camptothecin analogue 9-nitro-camptothecin (RCO.1), with that of its parental cell line. One hundred eighty-one genes, many of which known to be involved in nuclear factor κB and transforming growth factor β signaling and apoptosis, were found to be significantly overexpressed in the resistant compared with the parent line. However, many of the expression differences observed for apoptosis-related genes were in the direction "contrary" to that expected given the resistance of RCO.1. In other words, many of the genes found to be overexpressed in drug resistant-cells code for proteins promoting apoptosis. This finding led the authors to hypothesize a 2-step mechanism for the development of drug resistance. The first step would involve a decrease in apoptotic susceptibility through expression changes in the Bcl-2 and caspase gene families, and also in antiapoptotic pathways operating through Akt/PKB. The second step would involve changes in genes (including, in the case of this particular study, some genes in the nuclear factor κB and transforming growth factor β pathways) that can facilitate apoptosis but that would also promote cell proliferation in the presence of the drug.

A similar approach was used with paclitaxel, a microtubule stabilizing drug used to treat ovarian, breast and nonsmall cell lung cancer. Lamendola and coworkers[35] generated three sublines of the SKOV-3 human ovarian carcinoma cell line selected to represent early, intermediate, and late paclitaxel resistance. The expression profile of each of the four cell lines (parental SKOV-3 and the three resistant lines) was then determined by a cDNA array of ~9,600 known human genes. Early paclitaxel resistance phenotype was characterized by a sustained increase in expression of various genes encoding inflammatory proteins. Intermediate paclitaxel resistance was associated with overexpression of a significant number of extracellular genes, transport genes, and G1-S transition genes. Finally, late drug resistance was associated with an increase in expression of several tumor antigen, signal transduction, and plasma membrane genes.

More recently Kang and coworkers[36] examined by oligonucleotide microarrays genes that were differentially expressed in 5-FU-, doxorubicin-, and cisplatin-resistant gastric cancer cell lines, as compared with their drug-sensitive parent cell lines. These researchers identified over 250 genes differentially expressed in drug-resistant cell lines. They also identified eight genes that were associated with resistance to two or three of the tested drugs representing, therefore, possible candidate multidrug-resistance genes in gastric cancer.

The studies described above demonstrate that the gene expression changes acquired during the development of drug resistance are numerous and quite complex. In particular, it is not entirely clear whether all the changes acquired are required or whether only a few of genes are key to resistance and the others showed altered expression by coincidence, e.g., as a result of a cotranscriptional regulation.

Gene Expression Profiling of Clinical Tumor Samples

The identification and measure of expression of genes governing the sensitivity/resistance of tumors to anticancer drugs in clinical samples may, in principle, allow both prediction of the response of individual tumors and the selection of the most appropriate single drug or drug combination. As stressed by Winegarden,[37] the use of microarrays for predicting patient outcome has two major advantages compared with the use of single markers: (a) microarrays permit the screening of multiple genes without a-priori knowledge of which genes might be predictive; and (b) with microarrays it is possible to identify groups of genes, rather than single genes, that when analyzed together, may be a more reliable indicator of clinical outcome.

To date, only few clinical studies have attempted to correlate the response to chemotherapy of a tumor with its overall gene expression profile. Kihara and colleagues[38] profiled oesophageal tumors from patients who were to receive cisplatin/5-FU treatment and developed a drug response score based upon 52 genes each of whose level of expression was correlated with survival and thus, possibly, response to the anticancer drugs. This drug response score was shown to accurately predict survival in six independent patient samples.

A similar study from Okutsu and coworkers[39] used a cDNA microarray with the aim to predict the response of acute myeloid leukemia patients to chemotherapy (a combination o cytosine-arabinoside for 7 days and idarubicin for 3 days). Twenty-eight genes showed different expression levels in good responders (defined as subject achieving complete remission after one course of therapy) and poor responders (defined as subject not achieving complete remission after two courses of therapy). Using the expression data of these 28 genes, the authors established an algorithm to calculate a "drug response score" to predict individual clinical responses to chemotherapy. Interestingly, among 44 cases with positive drug-response scores, 40 achieved complete remission after treatment, whereas only 3 of 20 cases with negative scores responded well to the treatment.

Chang and collegues[40] profiled for gene expression core biopsy samples taken from 24 patients with primary breast tumors before neoadjuvant treatment (i.e., treatment before surgery) with docetaxel. Ninety-two genes were differentially expressed in tumors from patients that were sensitive or resistant to neoadjuvant chemotherapy. Using this molecular signature the authors could correctly classify 10 of 11 sensitive tumors and 11 of 13 resistant tumors.

More recently Ayers and coworkers[41] assessed whether gene expression profiling in breast cancer, at the time of diagnosis, could predict pathologic complete remission (defined as no histopathologic evidence of any residual invasive cancer cell in the breast) in response to neoadjuvant sequential weekly paclitaxel and 5-FU, doxorubicin and cyclophosphamide chemotherapy. A gene signature including 74 genes was identified, and found to be predictive of response (pathologic complete response or residual disease) with an overall predictive accuracy of 78% (14 of 18).

The results of the above-mentioned studies suggest that gene expression profiling of clinical tumor samples might greatly benefit cancer patients allowing a classification of tumors according to sensitivity or resistance to a chemotherapy regimen, thus preventing patient exposure to useless toxicity. However, a meta-analysis of 84 studies concerning prediction of various clinical cancer outcomes (death, metastasis, recurrence, response to therapy) by DNA microarrays revealed that the predictive performance of this technique is still quite variable.[42] The authors conclude that "larger studies with appropriate clinical design, adjustment for known predictors, and proper validation are essential for this highly promising technology".

Conclusions

Identifying the determinants of tumor sensitivity or resistance to anticancer drugs is still a challenge for the improvement of cancer chemotherapy. Since late '70s many cellular mechanisms of drug resistance have been identified by in vitro selection of anticancer drug-resistant clones, but it remains to be demonstrated whether they play a dominant role in clinical resistance. Recently, attempts to identify genetic determinants governing tumor chemosensitivity and to predict clinical response to chemotherapy have been made using the DNA microarray technology. Due to the multifactorial nature of cellular resistance to anticancer drugs, the use of DNA arrays in genome-wide analysis of cancer represent one of the most rational approaches to the discovery of predictive markers of treatment outcome in oncology, and to the identification of genes that determine tumor chemosensitivity.

References

1. Giaccone G. Clinical perspectives on platinum resistance. Drugs 2000; 59(Suppl 4):9-17, (discussion 37-18).
2. Pluen A, Boucher Y, Ramanujan S et al. Role of tumor-host interactions in interstitial diffusion of macromolecules: Cranial vs. subcutaneous tumors. Proc Natl Acad Sci USA 2001; 98(8):4628-4633.
3. Jain RK. Delivery of molecular and cellular medicine to solid tumors. Adv Drug Deliv Rev 2001; 46(1-3):149-168.
4. Dalton WS. The tumor microenvironment as a determinant of drug response and resistance. Drug Resist Updat 1999; 2(5):285-288.
5. Broxterman HJ, Lankelma J, Hoekman K. Resistance to cytotoxic and anti-angiogenic anticancer agents: Similarities and differences. Drug Resist Updat 2003; 6(3):111-127.
6. Dalton WS. The tumor microenvironment: Focus on myeloma. Cancer Treat Rev 2003; 29 (Suppl 1):11-19.
7. Muerkoster S, Wegehenkel K, Arlt A et al. Tumor stroma interactions induce chemoresistance in pancreatic ductal carcinoma cells involving increased secretion and paracrine effects of nitric oxide and interleukin-1beta. Cancer Res 2004; 64(4):1331-1337.
8. Gottesman MM, Fojo T, Bates SE. Multidrug resistance in cancer: Role of ATP-dependent transporters. Nat Rev Cancer 2002; 2(1):48-58.
9. Tew KD. Glutathione-associated enzymes in anticancer drug resistance. Cancer Res 1994; 54(16):4313-4320.
10. Poruchynsky MS, Giannakakou P, Ward Y et al. Accompanying protein alterations in malignant cells with a microtubule-polymerizing drug-resistance phenotype and a primary resistance mechanism. Biochem Pharmacol 2001; 62(11):1469-1480.
11. Gorre ME, Mohammed M, Ellwood K et al. Clinical resistance to STI-571 cancer therapy caused by BCR-ABL gene mutation or amplification. Science 2001; 293(5531):876-880.
12. Weisberg E, Griffin JD. Resistance to imatinib (Glivec): Update on clinical mechanisms. Drug Resist Updat 2003; 6(5):231-238.
13. Sartorius UA, Krammer PH. Upregulation of Bcl-2 is involved in the mediation of chemotherapy resistance in human small cell lung cancer cell lines. Int J Cancer 2002; 97(5):584-592.
14. Bignami M, Casorelli I, Karran P. Mismatch repair and response to DNA-damaging antitumour therapies. Eur J Cancer 2003; 39(15):2142-2149.
15. Shah MA, Schwartz GK. Cell cycle-mediated drug resistance: An emerging concept in cancer therapy. Clin Cancer Res 2001; 7(8):2168-2181.
16. Alaoui-Jamali MA, Dupre I, Qiang H. Prediction of drug sensitivity and drug resistance in cancer by transcriptional and proteomic profiling. Drug Resist Updat 2004; 7(4-5):245-255.
17. Karp JE. MDR modulation in acute myelogenous leukemia: Is it dead? Leukemia 2001; 15(4):666-667.
18. Scherf U, Ross DT, Waltham M et al. A gene expression database for the molecular pharmacology of cancer. Nat Genet 2000; 24(3):236-244.
19. Staunton JE, Slonim DK, Coller HA et al. Chemosensitivity prediction by transcriptional profiling. Proc Natl Acad Sci USA 2001; 98(19):10787-10792.
20. Musumarra G, Condorelli DF, Scire S et al. Shortcuts in genome-scale cancer pharmacology research from multivariate analysis of the National Cancer Institute gene expression database. Biochem Pharmacol 2001; 62(5):547-553.
21. Blower PE, Yang C, Fligner MA et al. Pharmacogenomic analysis: Correlating molecular substructure classes with microarray gene expression data. Pharmacogenomics J 2002; 2(4):259-271.
22. Vekris A, Meynard D, Haaz MC et al. Molecular determinants of the cytotoxicity of platinum compounds: The contribution in silico research. Cancer Res 2004; 64(1):356-362.
23. Huang Y, Anderle P, Bussey KJ et al. Membrane transporters and channels: Role of the transportome in cancer chemosensitivity and chemoresistance. Cancer Res 2004; 64(12):4294-4301.
24. Dan S, Tsunoda T, Kitahara O et al. An integrated database of chemosensitivity to 55 anticancer drugs and gene expression profiles of 39 human cancer cell lines. Cancer Res 2002; 62(4):1139-1147.

25. Zembutsu H, Ohnishi Y, Tsunoda T et al. Genome-wide cDNA microarray screening to correlate gene expression profiles with sensitivity of 85 human cancer xenografts to anticancer drugs. Cancer Res 2002; 62(2):518-527.
26. Nakatsu N, Yoshida Y, Yamazaki K et al. Chemosensitivity profile of cancer cell lines and identification of genes determining chemosensitivity by an integrated bioinformatical approach using cDNA arrays. Mol Cancer Ther 2005; 4(3):399-412.
27. Moriyama M, Hoshida Y, Otsuka M et al. Relevance network between chemosensitivity and transcriptome in human hepatoma cells. Mol Cancer Ther 2003; 2(2):199-205.
28. Mariadason JM, Arango D, Shi Q et al. Gene expression profiling-based prediction of response of colon carcinoma cells to 5-fluorouracil and camptothecin. Cancer Res 2003; 63(24):8791-8812.
29. Wallqvist A, Rabow AA, Shoemaker RH et al. Establishing connections between microarray expression data and chemotherapeutic cancer pharmacology. Mol Cancer Ther 2002; 1(5):311-320.
30. Brown JM. NCI's anticancer drug screening program may not be selecting for clinically active compounds. Oncol Res 1997; 9(5):213-215.
31. Kudoh K, Ramanna M, Ravatn R et al. Monitoring the expression profiles of doxorubicin-induced and doxorubicin-resistant cancer cells by cDNA microarray. Cancer Res 2000; 60(15):4161-4166.
32. Watts GS, Futscher BW, Isett R et al. cDNA microarray analysis of multidrug resistance: Doxorubicin selection produces multiple defects in apoptosis signaling pathways. J Pharmacol Exp Ther 2001; 299(2):434-441.
33. Zhou Y, Gwadry FG, Reinhold WC et al. Transcriptional regulation of mitotic genes by camptothecin-induced DNA damage: Microarray analysis of dose- and time-dependent effects. Cancer Res 2002; 62(6):1688-1695.
34. Reinhold WC, Kouros-Mehr H, Kohn KW et al. Apoptotic susceptibility of cancer cells selected for camptothecin resistance: Gene expression profiling, functional analysis, and molecular interaction mapping. Cancer Res 2003; 63(5):1000-1011.
35. Lamendola DE, Duan Z, Yusuf RZ et al. Molecular description of evolving paclitaxel resistance in the SKOV-3 human ovarian carcinoma cell line. Cancer Res 2003; 63(9):2200-2205.
36. Kang HC, Kim IJ, Park JH et al. Identification of genes with differential expression in acquired drug-resistant gastric cancer cells using high-density oligonucleotide microarrays. Clin Cancer Res 2004; 10(1 Pt 1):272-284.
37. Winegarden N. Microarrays in cancer: Moving from hype to clinical reality. Lancet 2003; 362(9394):1428.
38. Kihara C, Tsunoda T, Tanaka T et al. Prediction of sensitivity of esophageal tumors to adjuvant chemotherapy by cDNA microarray analysis of gene-expression profiles. Cancer Res 2001; 61(17):6474-6479.
39. Okutsu J, Tsunoda T, Kaneta Y et al. Prediction of chemosensitivity for patients with acute myeloid leukemia, according to expression levels of 28 genes selected by genome-wide complementary DNA microarray analysis. Mol Cancer Ther 2002; 1(12):1035-1042.
40. Chang JC, Wooten EC, Tsimelzon A et al. Gene expression profiling for the prediction of therapeutic response to docetaxel in patients with breast cancer. Lancet 2003; 362(9381):362-369.
41. Ayers M, Symmans WF, Stec J et al. Gene expression profiles predict complete pathologic response to neoadjuvant paclitaxel and fluorouracil, doxorubicin, and cyclophosphamide chemotherapy in breast cancer. J Clin Oncol 2004; 22(12):2284-2293.
42. Ntzani EE, Ioannidis JP. Predictive ability of DNA microarrays for cancer outcomes and correlates: An empirical assessment. Lancet 2003; 362(9394):1439-1444.

CHAPTER 9

SNP and Mutation Analysis

Lu Wang,* Robert Luhm and Ming Lei

Abstract

Genetic variation and SNP analysis starts with generation of sequence-specific signal, followed by the collection of that signal. The final step is extensive data analysis, which starts with conversion of quantifiable raw data and ends up with identified SNPs, frequencies, and sometimes tissue-specific expression patterns (levels). In this chapter we describe and compare the mechanisms of signal generation of several representative SNP analysis platforms. DNA microarray no doubt has its advantage in applications involving the classification and identification of tumor classes, gene discovery, drug dependent transcription mechanisms, as well as prediction of drug response. PCR, xMAP, invader assay, mass spectrometry, and pyrosequencing, on the other hand, are alternative methods of genotyping employed following the large scale screening and discovery of genetic variations. In addition, they offer higher specificity and sensitivity in analysis of both genomic DNA, as well as RNA. By exploiting these technologies, correlative study of the effects of putative genetic variations on cells, tissue-specific and developmentally specific expression is possible. Of extreme value are the many forms of Mass Spectrometry in the areas of sensitive, early cancer diagnosis. Finally, microarray and xMAP are suitable for protein analysis. While protein array offers higher through-put, xMAP is more amendable to the native 3D structure of protein molecules.

Introduction

With the derivation of the sequence of the human genome and the rise of proteomics to its current level of significance, a more comprehensive understanding of variation at both the genetic and expressed level has resulted. By no means is our understanding complete, but significant steps forward have been achieved. It is widely accepted that approximately 0.1 percent of the 3.2 billion bases of the human genome contain sequence variation. These variations happen in the forms of single and multiple nucleotide substitutions, as well as insertions, deletions, frame shifts, trinucleotide repeat expansions, and gene deletion or duplications. Sequence variation associated with a phenotypic change, often characteristic of a particular human disease, is referred to as a mutation. Sequence variations not yet known to be associated with phenotypic changes, are termed polymorphisms. While more and more polymorphism is found to be associated with a phenotypic change, the distinction between a mutation and a polymorphic variation is becoming difficult to define.[1-4]

Single Nucleotide Polymorphisms (SNPs) are the most common type of genetic variation. SNPs are scattered throughout the genome in both coding and regulatory regions of genes. A SNP in the coding region can alter protein structure and function, whereas a SNP in regulatory regions can alter expression patterns of the affected gene. These changes can lead to disease

*Corresponding Author: Lu Wang—Pel-Freez Biologicals, Rogers, Arkansas 72756, U.S.A. Email: lwang@pelfreez.com

Microarray Technology and Cancer Gene Profiling, edited by Simone Mocellin.
©2007 Landes Bioscience and Springer Science+Business Media.

symptoms and are called mutations. The abundance of SNPs and their tendency to remain stable genetically make them excellent biological markers. SNP profiling may help scientists to identify the full collection of genes that contribute to the development of complex diseases, such as cancer, and ultimately help to study correlations between SNPs and precancerous conditions. Additionally, SNPs and drug resistance in chemotherapy, cancer susceptibility, and drug response are currently some of the areas of interest for medical scientists.[5]

Genetic variation and SNP analysis starts with the generation of sequence-specific signal followed by the collection of that signal. The final step is extensive data analysis, which starts with, conversion of quantifiable raw data and concludes with identification of the SNPs, their frequencies, and potentially tissue-specific expression patterns (levels). In this chapter we will describe and compare the mechanisms of signal generation of several representative SNP analysis platforms. As an attempt to provide a reference point for medical professionals in their cancer study design and choice of technology platforms, we will also address the strengths and weaknesses of these platforms for creating a clinically useful SNP assay.

Enzymatic Approach

Historically, the enzymatic approach was the first widely used method for the detection of allelic variants. This method is based on the gain or loss of restriction endonuclease functionality by either the creation or loss of a specific recognition site. Restriction fragment length polymorphism (RFLP) is PCR amplification of a fragment of interest followed by the subsequent digestion of the fragment with a restriction endonuclease.[6,7] Cleavase Fragment Length Polymorphism Analysis (CFLP) is based on secondary structure of the primary sequence of single-stranded fragments, and their cleavage by engineered structure-specific endonucleases.[8] Single strand conformation polymorphism (SSCP),[9] double strand conformation polymorphism (DSCP),[10] and reference strand mediated conformation analysis (RSCA),[11] make use of labeled primers in the amplification step of both the reference and the sample DNA. This approach allows the analysis of the cleaved heteroduplexes on systems for automated DNA sequencing with its resultant increase in throughput. All these approaches exploit electrophoresis to fractionate digested DNA fragments of different sizes or secondary structures. As technology advanced, these approaches were superceded to varying degrees by chromatographic methods for discrimination of these allelic variants. Denaturing high performance liquid chromatography (DHPLC), is one example.[9]

Currently, SNP assays primarily require PCR amplification from genomic DNA. The resultant amplicons are further analyzed to screen or characterize potential SNPS. These assays are typically based on either hybridization, enzymatic cleavage, or a combination of both. Some assays can generate readable sequence directly from complementary DNA strands. In any case, these assays are amenable to liquid or solid phases. Some of the characteristics of the various assays are: differing sensitivity, specificity, linearity, throughput, cost and the flexibility of combination with expression analysis of functional SNPs.

Polymerase Chain Reaction (PCR)

Traditionally, Sequence Specific Primer Polymerase Chain Reaction (SSP-PCR) has been used as a cost-effective method that utilizes the 3'-end discrimination properties of polymerases, primarily that of Taq DNA polymerase. The PCR amplicons are detected and size-discriminated using agarose gel as the end-point of the reaction. Newer technologies, including microfluidics,[12] allow accurate sizing and quantification of these amplicons. Now, real-time chemistries have been invented to allow detection of amplification early in the exponential phase, while the reaction is occurring. This invention has been widely used in the analysis of correlation of sequence variation to expression level alteration in cancer cells.[13,14]

Application of TaqMan technology is routinely used for the real-time PCR based SNP analysis assay.[15,16] Briefly, as Figure 1 illustrates, this method combines the 5'exo-nuclease activity of AmpliTaq® Polymerase with FRET (Fluorescent Resonant Energy Transfer),

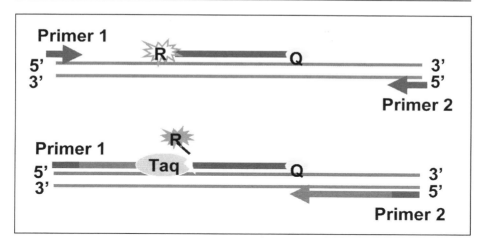

Figure 1. TaqMan probes. PCR primers 1 and 2 and a TaqMan probe, labeled with a fluorescent reporter dye "R", and a quencher dye "Q", bind to the DNA template. The 3' phosphate group prevents extension of the TaqMan probe. The presence of the enzyme, Taq polymerase, enables extension of the primer which displaces the TaqMan probe. The displaced probe is cleaved by Taq DNA polymerase resulting in an increase in relative fluorescence of the reporter. Polymerization is now complete.

making it possible to detect PCR amplification in Real-Time. The TaqMan® Probe is designed with a high-energy dye called a Reporter at the 5' end, and a low-energy molecule termed a Quencher at the 3' end. When this probe is intact and excited by a light source, the Reporter dye's emission is suppressed by the Quencher dye, due to the close proximity of the two dyes. If the probe is cleaved by the 5' nuclease activity of the enzyme, the distance between the Reporter and the Quencher increases thereby preventing energy transfer. The fluorescent emissions of the reporter increases while the quencher decreases. The increase in reporter signal is captured by the sequence detection instrument and integrated by the software. A significant advantage in this approach is that DNA or RNA analysis is performed in a gel free environment that is amenable to automation. More importantly, this offers enhanced sensitivity, specificity, and linearity resulting in the ability to detect two-fold changes in PCR quantity and an associated broad dynamic range.

Microarray Approaches

Microarray is a geometrically ordered array of biological material on a solid surface. It allows simultaneous data collection for detection and quantification of target material bound to probes on the solid surface. The signal generation method is primarily hybridization based in combination with enzymatic cleavage or extension of probes.[17] This technology now makes it possible to simultaneously consider the consequences of a myriad of genetic changes through the measurement of a large proportion of the complement of genes expressed in a given tissue at a given time.[18,19]

While DNA chips employ two-dimensional (2D) arrays of DNA molecules, a three-dimensional (3D) suspension array of microspheres offer a new approach to multiplexed assays for large-scale screening applications. Luminex® microspheres are polystyrene microspheres internally dyed with red and infrared fluorophores resulting in 100 optically distinct sets.[20] As Figure 2 illustrates, the DNA probe hybridization assays are configured in the same manner as current diagnostic assays for ease of use. Each bead set surface can be coated with oligonucleotides bearing a specific mutation sequence. Employing this approach, xMAP technology allows rapid and precise multiplexing of up to 100 unique assays within a

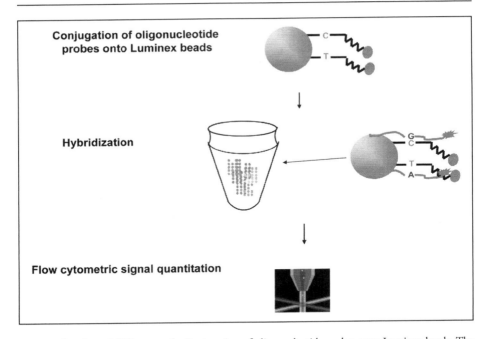

Figure 2. Luminex *x*MAP approach. Conjugation of oligonucleotide probes onto Luminex beads. The capture probes derived from SNPs of interests are coupled to different color-coded microspheres in separate reaction tubes. Conjugated beads are then mixed together for multiplexed hybridization assays. Phycoerythrin (PE)-conjugated streptavidin was added to the reaction to detect bound targets that were biotinylated. Each of reaction tube (well) contains up to 200 types of beads and one type of PCR amplicon. The signal of each target hybridized to its specific capture probe coupled to microspheres was determined by the fluorescence intensity of phycoerythrin. A reaction tube with all the components except the targets was used as a negative control. At least 200 microspheres of each set were analyzed by the Luminex[100] system.

single sample. Consequently bioassays can be developed that allow the capture and detection of specific analytes from a sample. Within the Luminex flow cytometry analyzer, lasers excite the internal dyes that identify each microsphere particle, as well as any reporter dye captured during the assay. Nucleic acids, proteins, lipids or carbohydrates can all serve as receptors to support the analysis of a wide range of biomolecular assemblies on Luminex microspheres. As a result, new applications in genomic and proteomic research are being continually developed and improved. Molecular analysis with microsphere arrays holds significant potential as a general platform for both research and clinical applications. This is due in part to recent innovations that provide for rapid serial analysis of samples. The technology is demonstrably superior in sensitivity, selectivity and throughput when compared to other available methodologies. By addition of alternative DNA probes, assays can be modified and enhanced thereby providing future expandability. Alternatively, intrinsic technical flexibility allows the use of reduced probe numbers effectively enhancing assay cost effectiveness when high degrees of multiplexing are unnecessary.[21,22]

Invader Assay

The Invader technology is a signal amplification system able to accurately quantify DNA and RNA targets with high sensitivity. In the invader reaction (Fig. 3), three single-stranded DNA chains form a ternary complex, the invasive structure, having a one base-pair overlap. This complex is composed of a DNA target molecule, which contains the SNP sequence of interest and two oligonucleotide sequences: an upstream invader and downstream probe. These

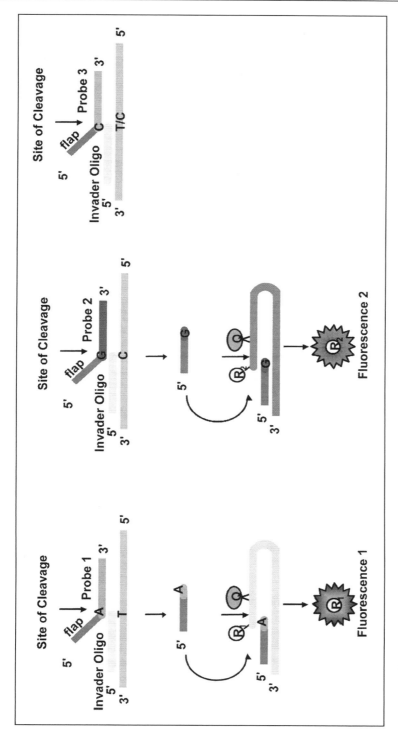

Figure 3. Mechanism of the Invader assay. Genotype 1 and Genotype 2 DNA form tripled stranded DNA structures and are recognized by the company's proprietary Cleavase enzyme. This leads to cleavage of the generic FRET probe and generation of a fluorescent signal. Genotype 3 does not form triple stranded DNA structures, the Cleavase enzyme will not recognize the structure, so no reaction takes place and no signal is generated.

three oligonucleotide strands hybridize to one another, forming a one base-pair junction causing the 5' end of the probe oligonucleotide to form a "flap". This structure is recognized and cut at a specific site by the Cleavase enzyme, thereby releasing the flap. The fragment now serves as the "Invader" oligonucleotide with respect to synthetic secondary targets and fluorescently labeled signal probes. The Cleavase enzyme subsequently cleaves the secondary signal probe generating a fluorescence signal. The detected signal is generated when this secondary probe, labeled with dye molecules capable of fluorescence resonance energy transfer, is cleaved. This event allows donor fluorescence to be detected with concomitant monitoring in real-time. If an incorrect DNA structure forms, the Cleavase enzyme will not recognize the structure, so no reaction takes place and no signal is generated.[23] Exquisite specificity is achieved by combining hybridization with enzyme recognition, providing discrimination of mutant from wild type at ratios greater than 1/1000 (mutant/wt). The technology is isothermal and flexible and incorporates homogeneous fluorescence readout. It is therefore readily adaptable for use in clinical reference laboratories, as well as high-throughput applications using 96-, 384-, and 1,536-well microtiter plate formats. Direct analysis of unamplified human genomic DNA to detect mutations and single-nucleotide polymorphisms is achievable. This characteristic provides the additional benefit of the eliminating many of the precautions requisite with preliminary amplification prior to analysis.

SNPs exhibit the potential to be present in four possible forms, or alleles, since DNA is synthesized from four different bases. But in reality, most SNPs are found consisting of just two alleles. An illustrative example is the case of the prothrombin G20210A mutation. In this case some people have a guanine at a base pair 20210 while others have an adenine at this genomic position. The possible cytosine and thymidine residues do not exist. The SNP in question is G/A restrictive.

A major advantage of the invader assay is its sensitivity, as demonstrated by the ability to score SNPs on nonamplified genomic DNA. It has been shown that the cleavage rates are 300 times higher when the probe sequence is complementary at the polymorphic base than when it is not. This precludes the possibility of false readings and confusion from contamination, which can occur during PCR. The invader assay is a method of SNP scoring that can eliminate the need for amplification of sample DNA and has been shown to work effectively in multiplexed assay formats.[24] In addition, it can also be used to quantify RNA amount.[25]

Mass Spectrometry

An extremely valuable technology in the area of sensitive early cancer diagnosis is mass spectrometry in its many forms. Cancer detection through the identification of proteomic patterns by surface-enhance laser desoption/ionization (SELDI) and electron spray ionization (ESI) mass spectrometry are finding greater acceptance. Instead of examining a patient for a single marker, a pattern of signals are analyzed within a mass spectrum to detect subtle variations. This holds promise for earlier detection with much greater sensitivity. Advancement such as these have been facilitated by the ever increasing sophistication of MS instrumentation and the analysis software employed to analyze the derived data. Although the products analyzed are typically low molecular weight, the utility of the method has been established. MS has the promise of high throughput and low cost routine analysis.[26,27]

Mass spectrometry has also been used successfully in the detection of low level amounts of DNA in patients with various cancers resulting from human papilloma virus infection.[28] In this case, the mode of mass spectrometry employed was matrix-assisted laser desorption/ionization time-of-flight (MALDI-TOF) coupled with real time competitive PCR and primer extension. This methodology allowed the accurate identification of HPV types 16 and 18 which are known to be high risk variants for the development of carcinomas. MALDI-TOF MS has been utilized for automated genotyping of SNPs using the simplified GOOD assay. In this particular approach, a single tube, purification free, three step approach is employed. Through the exploitation of PCR, primer extension and phosphodiesterase II digestion, immediate MALDI analysis is possible. The process is thereby amenable to automation.[29]

MALDI-TOF MS has been successfully utilized to quantify alternative splicing events in human pre-mRNA.[30] Alternative splicing has been suggested to occur in multi exonic genes with frequencies as high as 74%. The effects of improper alternative splicing have been linked to diseases such as cystic fibrosis, Parkinson's, Alzheimer's, and every major cancer. A rapid, reliable, and sensitive method of detecting and monitoring the occurrence and effects of alternative splicing defects has far reaching significance.

Sequencing

The current routine clinical method for DNA sequencing takes advantage of the dideoxy chain termination reaction.[31] The basis of this approach is dependant upon the controlled interruption of the enzymatic replication of a ssDNA template by DNA polymerase incorporation of dideoxynucleotide terminators. The base sequence of DNA is determined by fragmenting the genome (typically from a PCR product) into relatively short segments by virtue of the Sanger reaction. This produces a "ladder" of template-complementary DNA fragments that differ in length by one base pair and that bear unique fluorescent labels according to their terminal nitrogenous base. The fragments are electrophoretically separated on the basis of chain length. Single-base resolution is achieved through detection of base-specific labels, which are ultimately reassembled by base calling software. Through complex algorithms, the sequence of each fragment is reassembled into its original order. Electrophoretic DNA separation is almost exclusively carried out in a polymeric sieving matrix to exploit the molecules constant charge-to-frictional coefficient ratio. As a result, DNA separation in an electrophoretic field is independent of size other than direct size to mass. This sieving matrix can be either a cross-linked gel or an entangled polymer solution. A read length of 800 bases can typically be achieved although this depends on the length of the matrix, density of the matrix, and transit time through the matrix. In most cases, these factors can be varied to achieve the desired effect. A developmental goal of existing and future sequencing technology is the achievement of high-resolution DNA separations with extended read length that is both robust and low cost. By extending the read length of each single electrophoretic separation, the cost for de novo DNA sequencing can be reduced substantially. This subsequently reduces the number of templates required to sequence DNA contigs at a given redundancy and final sequence assembly will be faster, cheaper, and easier.[31-33]

In a Sanger sequencing reaction, nucleotide incorporation proceeds simultaneously along all DNA templates. This intrinsically generates sequence based typing (SBT) cis/trans ambiguities (Fig. 4, upper panel). Pyrosequencing is a real-time sequencing by synthesis method.[34,35] The mechanism of pyrosequencing™ is depicted in Figure 5. After a primer is hybridized to a single stranded DNA template, it is incubated in solution with the kinetically balanced enzymes, DNA polymerase, ATP sulfurylase, luciferase and apyrase. Additional reaction constituents include the substrates adenosine 5' phosphosulfate (APS) and luciferin. Each of the four deoxynucleotide triphosphates (dNTPs) is then individually added to the reaction mixture. When a dNTP is complementary to the base in the template strand, DNA polymerase catalyzes its incorporation into the DNA strand. Each incorporation event is accompanied by release of pyrophosphate (PPi) in a quantity equimolar to the amount of nucleotide incorporated. As the process continues, the complementary DNA strand is sequentially synthesized and the nucleotide sequence is determined from the signal peak in the pyrogram. One advantage that pyrosequencing has over sanger sequencing is that it can resolve cis/trans ambiguities in heterozygous DNA samples. Programmed sequential nucleotide incorporation makes pyrosequencing fundamentally different from the Sanger sequencing reaction. To pyrosequence an unknown DNA sequence, a cyclic nucleotide dispensation order (NDO) is generally used. As a result of each cycle of dATP, dGTP, dCTP and dTTP dispensation, one of the four dNTPs is incorporated into the DNA template while the other dNTPs are degraded by apyrase. When the DNA sequence is known, unique noncyclic NDOs can be programmed that generate sequence-specific pyrograms. Nucleotide incorporation along homozygous templates is always in-phase, whereas it can be either in-phase or out-of phase along heterozygous

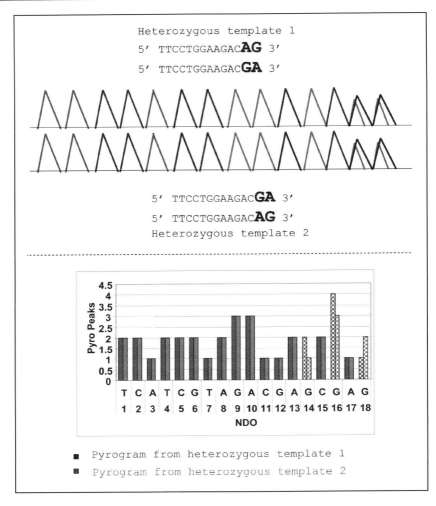

Figure 4. Comparison of Sanger sequencing and pyrosequencing. The upper panel illustrates intrinsic ambiguity at the two 3' end positions between two heterozygous templates. Red peaks represent T, blue peaks represent C, black peaks represent G, and green peak represent A. The lower panel illustrates that the nucleotide dispensation order, T(1st dispensation)CATCGTAGACGAGCGAG(18th dispensation) generates different programs from the same two heterozygous templates. In particular, the 14th, 16th, and 18th dispensations results in different numbers of nucleotide incorporation onto the two DNA templates. A color version of this figure is available online at www.Eurekah.com.

templates. When nucleotide incorporation into one allele is ahead of the other allele due to sequence polymorphisms, the pyrosequencing reaction goes out of phase. Each pyrogram peak represents the sum of nucleotide incorporation into DNA templates at the same or different but sequential base pair positions. This feature can be used to resolve SBT ambiguities.[36] As shown in the lower panel of Figure 4, the same numbers of nucleotides are incorporated into each pair of heterozygous templates until position 14, where out-of-phase nucleotide incorporation at the polymorphic positions result in different numbers of nucleotides incorporated, resulting in different peak heights. As nucleotide dispensation continues, uneven numbers of

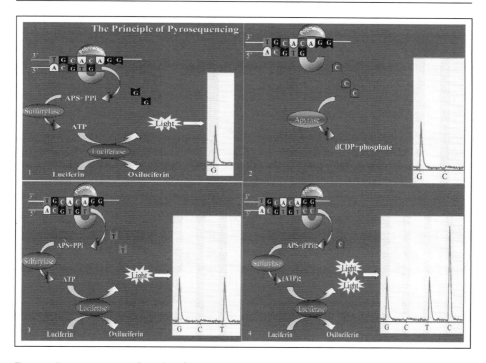

Figure 5. Pyrosequencing. The order of dNTP dispensation is programmed to be G (1st) C (2nd) T (3rd) C (4th). A pyrosequencing™ reaction mixture contains DNA polymerase, ATP sulfurylase, luciferase, apyrase, adenosine 5' phosphosulfate (APS) and luciferin. A sequencing primer is hybridized to a homozygous DNA template. 1) The first programmed dNTP dispensation event-dispensation of dGTP. DNA polymerase catalyzes the incorporation of the deoxynucleotide triphosphate G into the DNA strand. This is accompanied by release of pyrophosphate (PPi) in a quantity equimolar to the amount of incorporated nucleotide. ATP sulfurylase then quantitatively converts PPi to ATP in the presence of adenosine 5' phosphosulfate. This ATP drives the luciferase-mediated conversion of luciferin to oxyluciferin that generates visible light in amounts that are proportional to the amount of ATP. The light produced in the luciferase-catalyzed reaction is detected by a charge coupled device (CCD) camera and seen as a peak in a pyrogram™. The peak height represents the intensity of light signal, which is proportional to the number of nucleotides incorporated. Unincorporated dGTPs and excess ATP are degraded by apyrase. This sets a starting point for addition of another dNTP. 2) The second programmed dNTP dispensation event-dispensation of dCTP. Since cytidine is not complementary to adenosine in DNA template, dCTP is completely degraded by apyrase, generating no pyrogram™ peak. 3) The third programmed dNTP dispensation event-dispensation of dTTP. One single pyrogram™ peak is generated as a result of one nucleotide incorporation event. Unincorporated dTTPs and excess ATP are degraded by apyrase. 4) The fourth programmed dNTP dispensation event-dispensation of dCTP. Two pyrogram™ peaks are generated as a result of two nucleotide incorporation events. Unincorporated dCTPs and excess ATP are degraded by apyrase. Reprinted from reference 37, with permission.

nucleotide incorporation occurs at positions 16 and 18, resulting once again in different peak heights. By tailoring pyrosequencing NDO, virtually all SBT ambiguities can be resolved.[36] Other than significantly reducing cis/trans ambiguities, pyrosequencing offers additional advantages over sequencing. Among these are: (1) high laboratory efficiency resulting from the elimination of the electrophoresis step; (2) the capacity for relatively quantitative RNA expression analysis, and; (3) sequencing primer position flexibility coupled with immediate nascent sequence determination directly from the 3' end of the primer. With its compatibility with

Table 1. Comparison of approaches for mutation and SNPs analysis

Method	Mechanism	PCR Requirement	Detection	Application(s)
PCR				
AS-PCR (SSP)	Sequence or allele-specific-PCR	PCR	Gel-based and non-gel based end point read TaqMan, Homogeneous fluorescence	Genotyping
Real time PCR	5' nuclease assay	PCR, RT-PCR		Genotyping, mRNA quantification
Hybridization				
Microarray	Solid phase based	PCR	Fluorescence	Genotyping, mRNA quantification, protein quantification, Genotyping
Invader	Allele-specific hybridization with novel signal-amplification technology	+/-PCR, +/-RT-PCR	End point or real time fluorescence detection	mRNA quantification
Mass spectrometry	Mass differentiation of single or a number analytes	PCR, RT-PCR	Mass spectrometry	Diagnostics, expression profiling, novel gene identification
Sequencing				
Sequencing	PCR, RT-PCR	+PCR	Slab gel or capillary florescence	Genotyping, sequencing
Pyrosequencing	Sequencing by synthesis	+PCR	Light	Genotyping

robotic devices and automated dNTP dispensation, pyrosequencing provides an effective complementary tool for sequencing and hybridization based SNP analysis systems. Currently, the drawback of pyrosequencing is that is still reads short sequences as compared to standard sequencing, and its reagent costs are still on the high end.[37]

Summary

Table 1 compares the genetic variation analysis approaches described above. DNA microarray no doubt has its advantage in applications involving the classification and identification of tumor classes, gene discovery, determining drug affected transcription mechanisms, and in predicting drug response. PCR, xMAP, invader assay, mass spectrometry, and pyrosequencing, on the other hand, are genotyping alternatives performed following the large scale screening and discovery of genetic variations. In addition, they offer higher specificity and sensitivity in analysis of both genomic DNA, and RNA. By exploiting these technologies, correlative study of cell, tissue-specific and developmentally specific expression of genetic variation is possible. Of extreme value are the many forms of Mass Spectrometry in the areas of sensitive, early cancer diagnosis. Finally, microarray and xMAP are suitable for protein analysis. While protein array offers higher throughput, xMAP is more amendable to the native 3D structure of protein molecules.

References

1. Wang DG, Fan JB, Siao CJ et al. Large-scale identification, mapping and genotyping of single-nucleotide polymorphisms in the human genome. Science 1998; 280:1077-1082.
2. Cooper DN, Ball EV, Krawczak M. The human gene mutation database. Nucleic Acids Res 1998; 26:285-287.
3. Ng PC, Henikoff S. Accounting for human polymorphisms predicted to affect protein function. Genome Res 2002; 12:436-446.
4. Collins FS, Brooks LD, Chakravarti A. A DNA polymorphism discovery resource for research on human genetic variation. Genome Res 1998; 8:1229-1231.
5. The International SNP Map Working Group: A map of human genome sequence variation containing 1.42 million single nucleotide polymorphisms. Nature 2001; 409:928-933.
6. Lander ES, Botstein D. Strategies for studying heterogeneous genetic traits in humans by using a linkage map of restriction fragment length polymorphisms. Proc Natl Acad Sci 1986; 83(19):7353-7357.
7. Quan F, Korneluk RG, MacLeod HL et al. An RFLP associated with the human catalase gene. Nucleic Acids Res 1985; 13(22):8288.
8. Sander, Olson TS, Hall J et al. Comparison of detection platforms and post-polymerase chain reaction DNA purification methods for use in conjunction with Cleavase fragment length polymorphism analysis. Electrophoresis 1999; 20:1131-1140.
9. Gross E, Arnold N, Goette J et al. A comparison of BRCA1 mutation analysis by direct sequencing, SSCP and DHPLC. Hum Genet 1999; 105(1-2):72-78.
10. Arguello JR, Little AM, Pay AL et al. Mutation detection and typing of polymorphic loci through double-strand conformation analysis. Nat Genet 1998; 18(2):192-194.
11. Arguello JR, Little AM, Bohan E et al. High resolution HLA class I typing by reference strand mediated conformation analysis (RSCA). Tissue Antigens 1998; 52(1):57-66.
12. Panaro NJ, Yuen PK, Sakazume T et al. Evaluation of DNA fragment sizing and quantification by the agilent 2100 bioanalyzer. Clin Chem 2000; 46(11):1851-1853.
13. Shi C, Eshleman SH, Jones D et al. LigAmp for sensitive detection of single-nucleotide differences. Nat Methods 2004; 1(2):141-147.
14. Hu N, Flaig MJ, Su H et al. Comprehensive characterization of annexin I alterations in esophageal squamous cell carcinoma. Clin Cancer Res 2004; 10(18Pt 1):6013-6022.
15. Holland PM, Abramson RD, Watson R et al. Detection of specific polymerase chain reaction product by utilizing the 5'----3' exonuclease activity of Thermus aquaticus DNA polymerase. Proc Natl Acad Sci 1991; 88(16):7276-7280.
16. Livak KJ. Allelic discrimination using fluorogenic probes and the 5' nuclease assay. Genet Anal 1999; 14(5-6):143-149.
17. Chee M, Yang R, Hubbell E et al. Accessing genetic information with high-density DNA arrays. Science 1996; 274:610-614.

18. Mocellin S, Wang E, Panelli M et al. DNA array-based gene profiling in tumor immunology. Clin Cancer Res 2004; 10(14):4597-606.
19. Wang E, Adams S, Zhao YD et al. A strategy for detection of known and unknown SNP using a minimum number of oligonucleotides applicable in the clinical settings. J Transl Med 2003; 1:4.
20. Gordon RF, McDade RL. Multiplexed quantification of human IgG, IgA, and IgM with the Flowmetrix system. Clin Chem 1997; 43:1799-1801.
21. Smith PL, Walker Peach CR, Fulton RJ et al. A rapid, sensitive, multiplexed assay for detection of viral nucleic acids using the FlowMetrix system. Clin Chem 1998; 44:2054-2060.
22. Aston CE, Ralph DA, Lalo DP et al. Oligogenic combinations associated with breast cancer risk in women under 53 years of age. Hum Genet 2005; 116(3):208-221.
23. Kwiatkowski RW, Lyamichev V, de Arruda M et al. Clinical, genetic, and pharmacogenetic applications of the Invader assay. Mol Diagn 1999; 4(4):353-364.
24. Lyamichev V, Neri B. Invader assay for SNP genotyping. Methods Mol Biol 2003; 212:229-240.
25. Allawi HT, Dahlberg JE, Olson S et al. Quantitation of microRNAs using a modified Invader assay. RNA 2004; 10(7):1153-1161.
26. Petricon EF, Liotta LA. SELDI-TOF-based serum proteomic pattern diagnostics for early detection of cancer. Curr Opin Biotechnol 2004; 15(1):24-30.
27. Conrads TP, Hood, BL, Issaq HJ et al. Proteomic patterns as a diagnostic tool for early-stage cancer: A review of its progress to a clinically relevant tool. Mol Diag 2004; 8(2):77-85.
28. Yang H, Yang K, Khafagi A et al. Sensitive detection of human papillomavirus in cervical, head/neck, and schistosomiasis-associated bladder malignancies. PNAS 2005; 102(21):7683-7688.
29. Sauer S, Gelfand DH, Boussicault F et al. Facile method for automated genotyping of single nucleotide polymorphisms by mass spectrometry. Nuclec Acids Res 2002; 30(5):e22.
30. McCullough RM, Cantor CR, Ding C. High-throughput alternative splicing quantification by primer extension and matrix-assisted laser desorbtion/ionization time-of-flight mass spectrometry. Nucleic Acids Res 2005; 33:(11)e99.
31. Sanger F, Nicklen S, Coulson AR. DNA sequencing with chain-terminating inhibitors. Proc Natl Acad Sci 1977; 74:5463-5467.
32. Adams SD, Krausa P, McGinnis M et al. Practicality of high-throughput HLA sequencing based typing. ASHI Quarterly 2001; 25:54-57.
33. Adams SD, Barracchini KC, Chen D et al. Ambiguous allele combinations in HLA Class I and Class II sequence-based typing: When precise nucleotide sequencing leads to imprecise allele identification. J Transl Med 2004; 2(1):30.
34. Ronaghi M, Uhlen M, Nyrén P. A sequencing method based on real-time pyrophosphate. Science 1998; 281:363-365.
35. Ronaghi M. Pyrosequencing sheds light on DNA sequencing. Genome Res 2001; 11:3-11.
36. Ramon D, Braden M, Adams S et al. Pyrosequencing™: A one-step method for high resolution HLA typing. J Transl Med 2003; 1:9.
37. Wang L, Marincola FM. Applying Pyrosequencing to HLA-typing. ASHI Quarterly 2003; 27:16-18.

CHAPTER 10

Cancer Development and Progression

Mei He, Jennifer Rosen, David Mangiameli and Steven K. Libutti*

Abstract

Cancer development and progression is a complex process that involves a host of functional and genetic abnormalities. Genomic perturbations and the gene expression they lead to, can now be globally identified with the use of DNA microarray. This relatively new technology has forever changed the scale of biological investigation. The enormous amount of data generated via a single chip has led to major global studies of the cellular processes underlying malignant transformation and progression. The multiplicity of platforms from different proprietors has offered investigators flexibility in their experimental design. Additionally, there are several more recent microarrays whose designs were inspired by the nucleotide-based technology. These include protein, multi-tissue, cell, and interference RNA microarrays. Combinations of microarray and other contemporary scientific methods, such as, laser capture microdissection (LCM), comparative genomic hybridization (CGH), single nucleotide polymorphism analysis (SNP) and chromatin immunoprecipitation (ChIP), have created entirely new fields of interest in the more global quest to better define the molecular basis of malignancy. In addition to basic science applications, many clinical inquiries have been performed. These queries have shown microarray to have clinical utility in cancer diagnosis, risk stratification, and patient management.

Cancer Development

Cancer development and progression is a complex process that involves a host of functional and genetic abnormalities. This can include epigenetic modifications such as, changes in DNA methylation and histone acetylation, as well as the development of genomic mutations and other insults that can lead to altered gene expression and overall cell function. Inquiries into the molecular mechanisms behind malignant transformation and metastatic progression, is the basis for the development of many new diagnostic and therapeutic strategies.

Cancer can be considered a "developmental disorder", because it involves a disruption in the normal development of cells, in terms of both differentiation and proliferation.[1] Cancer cells generally contain the full complement of bio-molecules that are necessary for survival, proliferation, differentiation, cell death, and expression of cell-type specific function. Unfortunately, these components of cellular function are altered in terms of their regulation. The first cell to exhibit growth disinhibition has entered a process known as tumor initiation. The process is generally thought to require at least two genetic alterations; these cause the cell to lose its ability to mitigate the functional defect and subsequently become immortal. If progeny cells survive, they may go on to develop a progressive clonal population which leads to the primary tumor. The initiation and progression of tumors can either involve loss of tumor suppressor

*Corresponding Author: Steven K. Libutti—Surgery Branch, National Cancer Institute, National Institutes of Health, Bethesda, Maryland, U.S.A. Email: libutti@mail.nih.gov

Microarray Technology and Cancer Gene Profiling, edited by Simone Mocellin.
©2007 Landes Bioscience and Springer Science+Business Media.

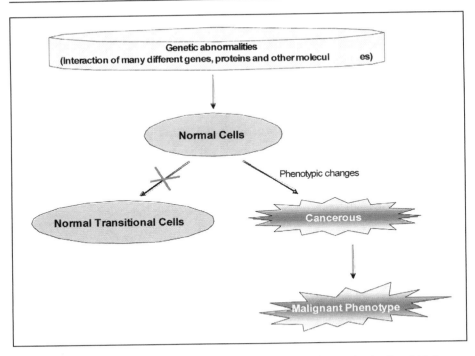

Figure 1. Genetic abnormalities cause phenotypic changes in normal transitional cells, which become cancerous and finally result in the "malignant phenotype".

function or induction of oncogene function, possibly both. The specific mechanisms that generate alterations in tumor suppressors and oncogenes vary among different tumor histologies and may even vary within the same histology for different patients. In some cases of soft-tissue sarcoma and papillary thyroid carcinoma, tumor initiation involves chromosomal rearrangements that activate various oncogenes.[2] This contrasts some colonic and pulmonary carcinomas, whereby initiation has been shown to involve oncogene and tumor suppressor alterations.[3]

The development of cancer exhibits several noteworthy phenomena. The first obvious behavior is the lack of normal constraint on cell proliferation. Cancer cells do not exhibit normal contact inhibition, in which cells proliferate until they reach a finite density, determined in part by the availability of certain growth factors. Transformed cells are often noted to survive in the absence of the growth factors that are normally required by their untransformed ancestors. This failure to undergo apoptosis during a state of deprivation has been postulated to contribute to the growth and survival of metastatic cells in ectopic sites. Instead of responding to the signals that cause normal cells to cease proliferation and enter the G_0 phase of the cell cycle, cancer cells continue to grow beyond the normal density limit. The tightly regulated processes that normally lead to senescence and apoptosis are grossly disrupted. Accumulation of these abnormalities contributes to the clinically relevant malignant phenotype (Fig. 1).

As additional mutations occur and the tumor progresses, there becomes a heterogeneous cell population. New phenotypes which portend lower rates of apoptosis, faster rates of division, lower metabolic requirements, increased ability to recruit neo-vasculature,[4] and metastatic competency gain a selection advantage and will ultimately assume a more dominant proportion of the tumor burden. This process of clonal selection continues as the disease progresses. Figure 2 is a summary of cancer development and progression.

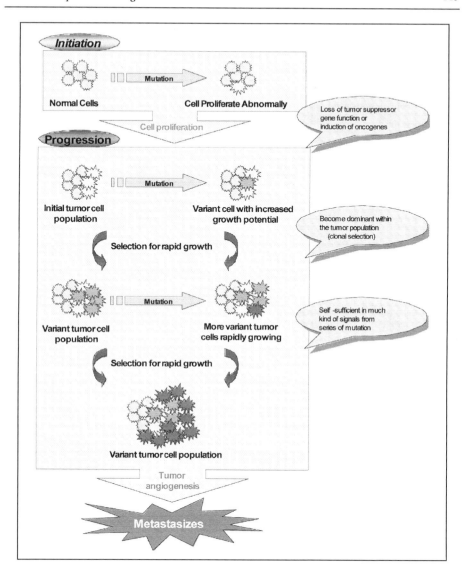

Figure 2. Process of cancer development. The development of cancer initiates when a single mutated cell begins to proliferate abnormally. Additional mutation followed by selection for more cells rapidly growing within the population then result in progression of the tumor to increasingly rapid growth and malignancy along with tumor angiogenesis.

There is evidence to suggest that significant genetic alterations may occur early in the natural history of a cancer.[5] The clinical correlation lies in the fact that the majority of cancers convey a prognosis which is anti-proportional to its stage at the time of detection. The rapidity of diagnosis and intervention is directly linked to survival. It therefore becomes quite obvious that a better understanding of tumorigenesis may not only lend itself to more sensitive screening techniques, but also may enable additional targeting of cancers, given their mechanisms of virulence. Owing to new technologies, the molecular picture of tumorigenesis and progression is unraveling and appearing to be a convoluted set of events within and between tumor cells and there surrounding tissue matrix.

Science/Technology

Microarrays

Genetic perturbations and the gene expression they lead to, can now be globally quantitated. Since the early 1990's, microarray technology has been successfully developed to give researchers the ability to measure tens of thousands of genes in parallel. It has caused a paradigm shift in the nature of investigation. Instead of hypothesis driven deduction, gene expression profiles between multiple groups can be screened for significant changes. Subsequently, genes of interest can be crossed with genes that displayed altered expression and the resulting subset can then enter validation and investigation. In the short history of this versatile technology, hundreds of large-scale experiments have been performed, generating global quantitative profiles of gene expression for multiple cancer histologies. Known types and subtypes of cancer have been readily distinguished by their gene expression patterns. More importantly, new molecular subtypes of cancer have been discovered that are associated with a host of tumor properties, including a tumor's propensity to metastasize and the sensitivity or resistance of a tumor to a particular therapy. The clinical utility of gene expression profiling is evidenced by recent investigations that show cancer gene expression signatures to potentially affect clinical decisions in the management of breast cancer and lymphoma.[6,7] It may not be long before all human cancers are profiled with a microarray gene chip, to ascertain a molecular diagnosis and prognosis, and define the optimal treatment strategy. The high-density array has been expanded to include protein microarrays,[8] carbohydrate microarrays,[9] multi-tissue microarrays,[10] cell microarrays[11] and small-molecule microarrays.[12] In this chapter, we will give a brief overview of some popular microarrays followed by a second section meant to convey clinical examples and implications.

DNA Microarray

One way of gaining information about tumorigenesis and progression is to identify genes whose expression is altered during the process. Traditionally, molecular inquiries into this have focused on relatively small numbers of genes or biomarkers. In so far as expression analysis, genes have generally been analyzed one at a time, by a variety of established methods including: northern analysis, nuclease-protection assays, reverse transcriptase-based primer extension, and RT-PCR. However, none of these approaches are readily amenable to increasing the volume of genes per inquiry, or "throughput". The advent of high-density DNA microarray technology provides a unique opportunity for high-throughput genetic analysis of tumor development,[13-15] and allows us to simultaneously visualize the expression of all genes within a cell population or tissue sample; hence, revealing its "transcriptome".

cDNA microarrays are ubiquitously used to evaluate differential gene expression. For two color array, two samples (typically a control and experimental sample) are used as sources of mRNA. After reverse transcription or during amplification, each of the samples is labeled with different fluorophores that have differing excitation frequencies. Both samples are then simultaneously allowed to hybridize to the microarray chip and the emission signals are read. The competitive binding of differentially labeled sources of transcript equivalents, provides an indirect, but internally controlled comparison of the mRNA levels corresponding to each arrayed gene. In contrast, Affymetrix based microarray is premised on sequence information alone. Chip sequences are synthesized in situ using a combination of photolithography and oligonucleotide chemistry. Oligonucleotides are synthesized as perfect match and mismatch pairs. These probe pairs allow the quantification and subtraction of signals caused by nonspecific cross-hybridization. The difference in hybridization signals between the samples, as well as their intensity ratios, serves as indicators of specific target abundance.

DNA microarray analysis can reveal correlations between the tumorigenicity of the cancer cells and changes in the expression levels of genes regulating cell growth, angiogenesis, and invasion. With primary analytic methods, such as multiple-hypothesis testing, use of clustering algorithms (groups genes and samples on the basis of expression profiles), and implementation of statistically based differential expression analysis (scores genes on the basis of their relevance to various clinical attributes), cancer types can be reliably distinguished from their normal tissues of origin. Predominant clinical and pathologic subtypes of cancer often have distinct gene expression profiles. Gene expression signatures of some primary tumors have been shown to predict disease recurrence, distant metastasis, survival and treatment response; however, this is still considered investigational. Cancers can be further sub-classified into molecular subtypes based on gene expression signatures. The changes in expression may provide insight into novel genes and pathways that are utilized in the progression and "dedifferentiation" of cancers.

Microarray technology is increasingly employed to establish expression profiles that may contribute to early cancer detection, and risk prediction and stratification. There is strong evidence that the aberrant genetic changes that occur with cancer progression, indeed happens at very early stages and remain persistent.[16-18] This lends itself to the plausible utility that microarray can be used as an adjunct method to clinicopathologic diagnostics, when results remains equivocal. Pathologic methods, which remain relatively limited to histology, histochemistry, and immunohistochemistry, may ultimately involve microarray as an adjunct technique or potentially as a validation step. Examples seen thus far come from both Lander and Staudt. Lander's group showed the ability of microarray to distinguish acute myeloid leukemia from acute lymphoblastoid leukemia,[19] whereas Staudt's group was able to further sub-classify diffuse large B-cell lymphoma into different categories.[20]

Microarray assembles and converges multiple other technologies, including automated DNA sequencing, mutational analysis, DNA amplification (PCR), oligonucleotide synthesis, nucleic acid labeling chemistries and bioinformatics. Aiding in this remarkable feat, DNA microarray has become the workhorse technique for gene expression studies. Fortunately, the many sources and widespread use of microarray technology have thus far allowed researchers to retain flexibility in their choice of platforms. The major platforms are summarized in Table 1.

Protein Microarrays

In light of the completion of the human genome project, DNA microarrays and bioinformatics platforms now give scientists a global view of biological systems. Proteomics is integral in advancing our understanding of disease processes, particularly because it can potentially identify protein biomarkers for diagnostic and therapeutic targeting. Protein profiling provides important information for tumor development since many changes associated with tumor progression may be post-transcriptional or post-translational. Genomic and proteomic research tools enable genome-wide assessment of gene expression and kinase driven cell signaling events. Within the last few years, microarray technology has expanded beyond DNA chips. Protein microarray techniques have already demonstrated that this technology is capable of filling the gap between genomics and proteomics. Protein microarray has become a key technology for proteome research[21,22] and has been applied to the identification, quantification and functional analysis of proteins. Some examples include the analysis of protein-DNA, protein-protein, protein-oligosaccharide, enzyme-substrate and protein-drug interactions.[23-25] Protein arrays contain a number of immobilized protein spots; proteins being antibodies, cell lysates or recombinant proteins. To determine the protein content, the arrays are incubated with a tagged unknown biologic sample or labeled antibody.[26] Similar to DNA microarrays that reveal the gene expression profile at the mRNA level, this approach is thought to provide a "snapshot" of the protein content of cells or tissues at a given time.

Table 1. Platforms of DNA microarrays

DNA Probe	Strength and Weakness
Robotically Spotted Presynthesized Probes:	
• PCR products of cDNA library clone inserts (One or two probes/gene) (Home-made or commercial)	Relatively inexpensive; flexibility in determining array content and coverage. Possibility of cross-contamination of cDNA clones/PCR products; it is difficult to obtain comprehensive coverage or specific sequences
• Long oligonucleotides (40-80-mer) (One probe/gene) (Printed in house, complex libraries from: ClonTech; MWG Biotech; Operon)	Relatively inexpensive; probe sequences and genes coverage is controllable; less chance of probe cross contamination and cross-hybridization with un-related sequences; more sensitive; changes or modifications are more straightforward.
In Situ Synthesized Arrays:	
• 25-mer oligonucleotides (multiple perfect and mismatch probes/gene) (Affymetrix, Inc. GeneChips)	Abroad of coverage; consistency; carefully designed standard operating procedures; the mismatch probe is used as a control to detect background noise and cross-hybridization from unrelated probes; Reproducibility and specificity are higher that other platforms. Cost is considerable; changes are not readily accommodated when new sequence information becomes available or if different arrays are desired.

Multi-Tissue Microarrays

Many genes and signaling pathways that control cell proliferation, differentiation, genomic integrity, and apoptosis are involved in cancer development. New techniques, such as serial analysis of gene expression and cDNA microarrays, have enabled measurement of the expression of thousands of genes in a single experiment, revealing many new, potentially important cancer genes. These genome screening tools can comprehensively survey one tumor at a time; however, analysis of hundreds of specimens from patients in different stages of disease is required to establish the diagnostic, prognostic and therapeutic importance of each gene candidate. Subsequent validation of the clinical value of such candidate genes or proteins requires large-scale analysis of human tissues, and tissue analysis by conventional strategies is slow and expensive. The recently developed array-based high throughput technique, termed multi-tissue microarray,[10] has overcome these limitations, allowing parallel molecular profiling of large numbers of samples. As many as 1000 tissue biopsies from individual tumors can be distributed in a single tumor tissue microarray. Sections of the microarray provides targets for multiple types of parallel analyses, including fluorescence in situ hybridization (FISH), RNA in situ hybridization (mRNA-ISH) and immunohistochemistry (IHC),[27] yielding the ability to detect DNA, RNA and protein targets in each specimen on the array. Additionally, consecutive sections allow the rapid analysis of hundreds of molecular markers in the same set of specimens. The benefits include: large number of cases can be assessed simultaneously for numerous markers, processing retains identical conditions, reduced levels of archival tissue, excellent correlation with standard methods, reduction in cost and time, and ability to establish associations between molecular changes and clinical endpoints.

Simultaneous hybridization of a single sample to thousands of different specified targets is become central to life-science research. With the genomic sequencing of dozens of species now complete, focus is shifting onto gene function. In a twist of canonical microarray technology, the transfected cell microarrays are another advance in the miniaturization and simplification of high-throughput assays in cultured mammalian and *Drosophila melanogaster* cells, (which the more direct tools of classical genomics have been difficult to implement). RNA interference (RNAi) microarray makes possible discrete, parallel transfection with thousands of RNAi reagents on a single microarray slide.[28] These capabilities are aiding the field of functional genomics, by making loss-of-function genetics more amenable in numerous organisms. The discovery of a gene-product that confers lethality when knocked-down could provide an inroad for new cancer therapies. The majority of the scientific-medical community believes that microarray technology will be routinely used in the selection, assessment, and quality control of drugs earmarked for development, as well as for diagnosis, risk prediction and response to therapy.

Complementary Approach

Laser Capture Microdissection

Many tissue samples contain heterogeneous cell populations. The specific cell line of interest may only represent a small percentage of the total tissue volume. To explore the molecular differences among distinct pathological stages of cancer, the pure populations of juxtaposed normal cells and interposed stromal cells must be separable from malignant cells. Laser capture microdissection (LCM) has provided an efficient and reliable one-step method for obtaining pure populations of cells from stained tissue sections under direct microscopy.[29,30] Select subpopulations are isolated by LCM without contamination from other cell types. LCM and the strategies premised on T7-based in vitro transcription for RNA amplification (T7- IVT),[31] PCR-based RNA amplification,[32] and DNA microarray,[18] facilitate gene expression profiling of pure cell populations. Several studies have shown that T7-IVT provides sensitive and minimally biased results for the detection of sample differences.[33,34] LCM has also made it possible to separate the contributions of expression changes from different locations within the same tumor.[35] It offers an opportunity to better resolve the dynamic relationship between the malignancy and its surrounding tissue matrix.

Comparative Genomic Hybridization

Genomic DNA copy number alterations are key genetic events in the development and progression of some human cancers. Tumors develop through the combined processes of genetic instability and survival-based selection, resulting in clonal populations that have accumulated the most advantageous set of genetic aberrations. Many types of instability may occur, including and resulting in point mutations, chromosomal rearrangements, alterations of microsatellite sequences and epigenetic changes. These abnormalities act alone or in combination, altering the functional levels of cellular products. Gene deletions, duplications and amplifications frequently contribute to tumorigenesis. Developmental abnormalities may also result from gain or loss of a chromosome or chromosomal region before or shortly after fertilization. This can result in a field defect of an organ or tissue which is at high risk to develop multiple primary tumors. Thus, detection and mapping of copy number abnormalities provides an approach for associating aberrations with disease phenotype and for localizing critical genes. Comparative genomic hybridization (CGH) was the first efficient approach to scanning the entire genome for variations in DNA copy number. CGH evaluates parallel changes in DNA copy number and subsequently gene expression for a given tumor sample, and allows analysis of the changes that accumulate during tumor progression.[36] Candidate genes in the regions of loss can be assessed as to whether there is altered expression, and the remaining copy can further be evaluated for genetic or epigenetic changes.[37] In a typical CGH measurement, differentially labeled total genomic experimental DNA and normal reference DNA are cohybridized to normal chromosome spreads or, more recently, DNA microarrays. The resulting ratios of fluorescent intensities along the length of chromosomes, at a location on the "cytogenetic map", are approximately proportional to the ratio of copy numbers for corresponding DNA sequences relative to the reference genome. Because the reference genome is normal, increases and decreases in the intensity ratio, directly indicate DNA copy-number discrepancies. Chronic lymphocytic leukemia was recently a backdrop for a clinical trial using CGH to define genomic aberrations as they portend to therapeutic efficacy.[38] Correlation of DNA copy-number aberrations with prognosis has been found in a variety of cancer histologies, including prostate,[39] breast,[40] gastric[41] and lymphoma.[42] Expression genomics is having a profound influence on providing correlative information that is clinically useful. There is optimism that these types of global methods, when used together, will lead to an advanced understanding of the malignant process and confer onto us the ability to abrogate their untoward outcomes.

Genome-Wide SNP Genotyping Assay

Common diseases, such as diabetes, cancer and heart disease, have both environmental and genetic implications. Although, any two unrelated people are about 99.9% genetically equivalent, understanding the remaining 0.1% is crucial, because it contains the genetic variants that influence how people differ in their risk to develop disease, as well as their response to treatment. Single nucleotide polymorphisms (SNPs) are sites in the genome, where a specific DNA sequence from many individuals differs by a single base pair. The human genome contains more than ten million common SNPs. A smaller number of select 'tagging' SNPs can be used to map the majority of genetic variations between individuals.[43] In fact, preliminary estimates indicate that ~200-300K tagging SNPs are required to map most of the variation in the genome.[44,45] It quickly becomes obvious that the development of microarray-based methods for SNP genotyping is a demanding task that is determined not only by SNP multiplexing, but also by the limiting number of samples that can be processed in parallel.[46] The robustness of the multiplexed microarray-based SNP genotyping systems is determined by the reaction principles applied for SNP allele distinction and the microarray formats used. In an optimal system, two oligonucleotides will hybridize only if they are completely complimentary in their base pair sequence.[47] If there is a single base pair mismatch then hybridization efficiency will suffer. Perfectly matched sequences hybridize more efficiently to their corresponding oligomers on the array, therefore giving stronger fluorescent signals over mismatched probe-target combinations. Oligonucleotide hybridization can therefore discriminate between the two alleles of an SNP. Microarrays contain large numbers of human SNPs. PCR amplification of genomic DNA followed by hybridization to arrays permits the detection of chromosomal regions that sustained loss of heterozygosity (LOH).[48,49] This provides an automated high-throughput method for large-scale LOH analysis. In addition, these high-resolution genotyping arrays are applicable to genomic profiling and allelic expression measurements. The microarray-based SNP methods have already found some medical applications. Several recent studies have found that SNP panels provide higher quality data, better genotyping accuracy, larger information content, and may also have a higher power to detect linkage, compared with panels of microsatellite markers.[50,51]

ChIP-on-Chip for Binding Partners

ChIP-on-Chip analysis is a microarray-based method for determining genome-wide transcription binding partners during specific biological processes[52] and location analysis of transcriptional regulatory networks that control cell cycle progression and differentiation.[53] ChIP-on-Chip, the combination of Chromatin Immunoprecipitation (ChIP) with microarray technology is an efficient method of identifying in vivo protein-DNA interactions. In this technique, cells are treated with a cross-linking reagent, which covalently links protein complexes to DNA. The cross-linked chromatin is isolated, fragmented, and subject to immunoprecipitation of the protein component. These proteins and attached DNA fragments are purified and undergo a lytic reversal of cross-linkage. The DNA fragments are labeled with a fluorescent dye and hybridized to a microarray chip, with probes corresponding to genomic regions of interest (ChIP-chip).[54] ChIP assays have the advantage of detecting transcription factor binding before gene activation, yielding the ability to evaluate the association of a specific transcription factor with their affiliated promoter or enhancer regions in the context of the native chromatin conformation.[55] The higher order structure of chromatin may allow the regulatory regions and transcription factors to come into close proximity, either by direct physical interactions or by interactions through bridging molecules.[56] Understanding how these proteins selectively bind to specific promoters may reveal new therapeutic strategies that allow the manipulation of cellular behavior in both normal and diseased states. This assay allows us to profile the kinetic behavior of transcription factors and other coregulatory elements, potentially thousands of regulatory regions at a time.

Nuclear Run-on Assay

The nuclear run-on assay is most commonly used to determine treatment-induced changes in relative rates of transcription, for specific genes. This assay measures changes in the number of active transcriptional complexes on a gene, which is generally accepted to be an index of transcriptional activity for that gene.[57] The combination of the nuclear run-on technique with microarray[58] provides an investigational approach which allows the simultaneous assessment of nuclear premRNA and cytoplasmic RNA. Thus, changes in gene expression can be examined at both the level of transcriptional regulation and transcript stabilization. Nuclear run-on is performed by isolating nuclear RNA, amplifying it with the incorporation of ^{32}P-UTP, and hybridizing it to nascent RNA transcripts on a microarray chip. This technique results in dynamic information that can explain the initial response of a cell to environmental stimuli, including pharmacologic exposure.

In Vitro/Preclinical Research Using Microarray

In order for tumors to grow beyond a small size or to metastasize, they must develop a supportive blood supply. Under normal circumstances, angiogenesis is the balanced formation of new blood vessels from preexisting ones, required for most bodily and cellular functions to occur. Angiogenesis occurs as a cascade of events that may become deregulated during abnormal tumor induction. Whether deregulation is the result of multiple early genomic insults or as aberrations in protein formation, folding and function is still unclear. The study of neovasculature is therefore an ideal model to apply microarray technology to better define the early expression changes and their sequelae.

Ideally, antiangiogenic therapy would target endothelial cells and block tumor angiogenesis specifically while allowing normal angiogenesis to occur. While there are many studies characterizing these inhibitory agents, the mechanisms of action remain unclear. Our laboratory has pursued an approach that combines the rational use of microarray technology with its complementary techniques to elucidate common pathways in angiogenesis and better understand the underlying mechanism of action of new antiangiogenic agents. As one example using cDNA microarrays along with siRNA and RT-PCR, Mazzanti et al[59] have recently investigated the early effects of two different antiangiogenic reagents on human endothelial cells: endostatin (an endogenous protein) and fumagillin (a exogenous compound and a natural metabolite from Aspergillus fumigatus). These reagents were incubated with endothelial cells over several time points up to 8 hours; a majority of gene expression changes were observed as early as one hour following treatment. Untreated endothelial cells were used as the experimental control. Interestingly, many of the genes altered early in treatment were involved with cell proliferation, gene transcription and matrix organization. Not unsurprisingly, a number of the other genes identified have no known function as of yet, but with further study may prove to be essential components of the cell's complex processes. Four genes had a similar expression profile for both agents over the time course studied: DOC1, KLF4, TC-1 and ID1. The changes in each of these selected genes were confirmed using real time quantitative RT-PCR and were analyzed for specificity on HUVEC cells by comparing these agents with 5FU over the same duration. Three of the genes had the same profile by TaqMan (DOC1, TC1 and KLF4) as seen in the microarray data. However, ID1 did not show any significant change by TaqMan, possibly due to cross-hybridization of the message for a similar gene with the ID1 spot. In comparison, no significant changes for these genes were seen over the course of treatment in fibroblasts. This suggests that these changes are unique responses of endothelial cells to endostatin and fumagillin. We further demonstrated that small interfering RNA (siRNA) to KLF4 and TC1 fails to upregulate in response to endostatin treatment when DOC1 was silenced. This suggests that DOC1 may be upstream to these two genes; since this abrogation did not occur following fumagillin treatment, we may surmise that the interactions among these genes is different depending on the antiangiogenic reagent and may lead to different downstream pathways. Further study of these genes and their complex regulatory system is ongoing.

In other work done in our laboratory, Feldman et al[60] used microarray technology to compare the effects of an angiogenesis inhibitor on gene expression profiles in vitro to those observed in vivo. Tissue inhibitor of metalloproteinase 2 (TIMP-2) is an angiogenesis inhibitor which was initially thought to exert its effect by blocking matrix metalloproteinases (MMPs). As is often the case, the translation from in vitro to in vivo clinical studies of synthetic small molecule inhibitors of MMPs has been disappointing. We hypothesized that the antiangiogenic activity of TIMP-2 may actually rely on MMP-independent mechanisms, and that manipulation of the tumor-host response can facilitate anticancer strategies. We developed a strategy combining microarray technology in order to compare both in vitro cultured cells and in vivo tumor following TIMP-2 overexpression in order to elucidate these pathways. Murine colon adenocarcinoma cells (MC38) were transduced with either an empty retrovirus or a retrovirus encoding human TIMP-2 and stable clones were produced. Interestingly, TIMP-2 overexpression resulted in inhibition of tumor growth in syngenic mouse xenografts but not in cell culture. MC38/TIMP-2 tumors were compared to in vitro culture on cDNA microarray in order to identify the genes involved in tumor-host interactions. Our selection criteria yielded thirteen candidate genes, based on their persistent expression differences in vivo that were not present in vitro. We chose Ptpn16, the murine analogue for human MKP-1, for further study based on the known relationship of this gene to TIMP-2 related processes in angiogenesis. Specifically, the MAPK pathway plays an important role in angiogenesis, and MKP-1 is a dual-specificity phosphatase implicated in its regulation. MKP-1 dephosphorylates p38 MAPK which mediates the angiogenic response to VEGF and bFGF. Using a new technique of multireplicate protein-blotting for tissue array, aka layered protein scanning, protein expression patterns were analyzed. MC38 transduced with TIMP-2 demonstrated a 2.8 fold increase in MKP-1 expression, a 34% decrease in p38 phosphorylation, and no changes in total p38 expression compared to null transduced tumors. However, the in vitro level of MKP-1 expression, between null and TIMP-2 transduced tumor cells, were similar. These findings suggest that there is a link between MKP-1 up-regulation and TIMP-2 induced inhibition of angiogenesis in vivo. We could accelerate the growth of MC38/TIMP-2 tumor when using orthovanadate, a phosphatase inhibitor, to treat animals bearing MC38/TIMP-2 xenografts. We could also completely reverse the TIMP-2 induced dephosphorylation of p38 in this manner. Adding TIMP-2 to the endothelial culture medium also resulted in a 2-fold increase in the amount of MKP-1 bound to MAPK. This supports our hypothesis that MKP-1 associated MAPK inactivation mediates the antiangiogenic effects of TIMP-2. By the use of microarray and its complementary techniques, these experimental approaches might elucidate molecular pathways that differ in vitro from in vivo, and therefore may be useful as a strategy for rational targeting for antiangiogenic therapy.

Clinical Studies

Microarrays and their complementary technology are not only important for basic science research, but also have many applications in clinical study of cancer. Earlier diagnosis of cancer either in situ or through circulating biomarkers could lead to more targeted treatments and better recurrence surveillance. More effective treatments of late-stage or metastatic disease could improve patient survival and overall quality of life. Better prediction of a patient's response to therapy, prior to treatment itself, could allow for more rational use of toxic anticancer agents. Ideally, we could even prevent cancer from forming by use of preventive agents in patients with either an inherent genetic predisposition to cancer or those in whom the earliest stages of neoplastic processes can be detected. Regardless of presumptive applications, it is clear that the interplay between bench and bedside is critical.

Gene Expression Signatures

There are many examples of the use of gene expression signatures in the prediction of benign versus malignant disease. Our laboratory has a significant interest in using microarray technology and its complementary techniques in the analysis of thyroid tumors. Diagnosis of thyroid disease currently remains based on the gold standard of fine needle aspiration biopsy. Up to 10-25% of these samples are read as indeterminate by histopathologic criteria, necessitating thyroid lobectomy for diagnosis. The identification of a gene expression signature that can determine a specific type of tumor could help solve this clinical dilemma. Recently, we developed a novel classification scheme for thyroid tumors that was able to accurately predict the likelihood of benign versus malignant disease based on microarray analysis using as few as six genes.[61] We built a predictor model using[62] samples from patients with four types of thyroid lesions: papillary thyroid cancer and follicular variant of papillary thyroid cancer for the malignant tumors; follicular adenoma and hyperplastic nodule for the benign disease. We chose these four types as they represent the majority of suspicious thyroid lesions.

We extracted the RNA, amplified it according to a modification of the standard Eberwine technique, and hybridized it along with its control to a cDNA microarray chip. We chose as an appropriate control a pooled reference standard of normal thyroid tissue. This is a replenishable source against which all samples and future samples can be analyzed. This way, we can compare gene changes from patient to patient. It is also important to note that the mRNA extracted from all samples and from the reference controls were amplified. Our lab and others have found that there is increased sensitivity without a loss of quality or resultant bias so long as the samples are amplified in a similar fashion.

Analysis of the overall gene expression profiles revealed that the benign lesions (FA, HN) could be distinguished from the malignant lesions (PTC, FVPTC) (Fig. 3). We used a statistical analysis program (Partek, Inc.) to discover two informative combinations of genes that to create a predictor model; one model contained six genes, and one contained a combination of 10 genes. We were able to correctly predict the diagnosis of all 10 unknown samples, with a more accurate prediction using the 6 gene combination. We were then able to design primer/probe pairs for RT-PCR to more precisely quantitate the differences in these gene expression patterns in our six gene model.[62] Again, we were able to correctly predict the diagnosis of 17 of 20 unknown samples. Interestingly, of the 11 genes that were informative for the diagnosis, five genes are known genes, and for the other six genes, no functional studies are yet available. In three of the genes, the pattern of expression by RT-PCR is very similar between the benign and malignant samples (Fig. 4). However, removing these genes from the analysis rendered us unable to properly diagnose our unknowns. Therefore, it is important to note that this type of analysis derives it power from the pattern of genes that are analyzed, rather than the degree of up or downregulation of any particular gene. In training the algorithm, the computer is not biased with any knowledge of genes previously associated with thyroid cancer; it simply identifies those genes that best differentiate the diagnostic groups. Any single gene found on univariate analysis to be associated with thyroid cancer may not turn out to be important in a multivariate

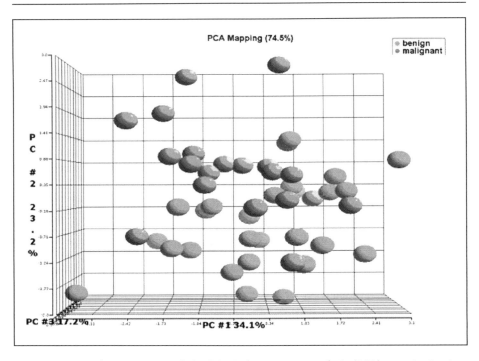

Figure 3. Principal component analysis. Principal component analysis (PCA) organization in a three-dimensional space of our group of 47 samples. Each sphere represents how that sample is localized in space on the basis of its gene expression profile across the six informative genes. The distance between any pair of points is related to the similarity between the two observations in high-dimensional space. The PCs are plotted along the three axes shown, x y and z. The percentage indicates the total amount of variance captured by the principal components; the first is the one capturing the largest amount of variance or information and so forth. Benign tumors include the diagnoses of hyperplastic nodule and follicular adenoma; malignant includes papillary thyroid carcinoma and follicular variant of papillary thyroid carcinoma.

predictor of diagnosis. This study is one clear example of how gene expression profiling can provide very useful diagnostic information; we expect it is highly likely that gene expression profiling will be incorporated in future studies for clinical decision making. This makes it very important to have a reproducible, well-established protocol for sample handling and replenishable, appropriate reference controls. Moving from the discovery phase using microarray to a more robust, affordable and commercially available testing system based on RT-PCR raises the hope that this is possible.

Similar predictor models have been developed that predict survival in colorectal cancer patients,[63] where microarray-based molecular staging based on 43 genes was better able to predict 36-month survival than traditional clinical staging. Other applications for microarray based gene expression signatures have been to identify the likelihood of a patient dying from cancer and therefore predict therapeutic failure in a variety of cancer types.[64] In this study, mouse and human comparative translational genomics were applied and identified an 11-gene signature that was characteristic for distant metastatic lesions in a transgenic mouse model of prostate cancer. This signature was then applied to a set of clinical samples from 1153 patients with eleven different types of cancer. Rigorous statistical analysis demonstrated that this expression profile could consistently predict a shortened interval to disease recurrence, distant metastasis and even death following therapy in these patients. According to the authors, this signature resembled a gene expression pathway essential for stem cell survival; they posit that

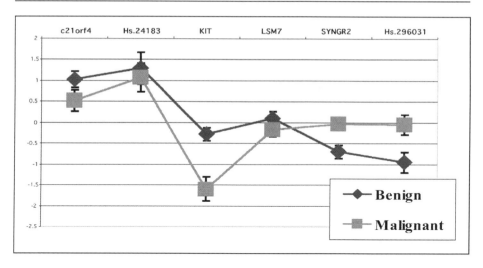

Figure 4. A graph showing gene expression profiles of all 47 samples used to train the class prediction rule. The y axis represents the ratio between normal thyroid mRNA expression and thyroid lesion mRNA expression of each of the genes converted to a log2ratio scale.

activation of these genes may promote tumor progression, accounting for the outcomes in this patient group.

In a related approach, Sanchez-Carbayo et al[65] used cDNA microarrays using both known genes and expressed sequence tags to identify relevant genes involved in bladder cancer progression and further validated several of these targets by immunohistochemistry and tissue microarray. Clustering yielded subgrouping within early-stage tumors that could be correlated with different overall survival.

Another technique for microarrays has been to fabricate novel, focused arrays from expressed sequence tags derived from the cell or tissue type of interest. In one example, a cDNA microarray for gastric cancer was created[66] and used to compare gene expression from human gastric cancer cell lines to a normal cell line. Further exploration of the forty differentially expressed genes was using reverse-transcription PCR, Western blotting and immunohistochemical staining. If the expression of these genes can in fact be coregistered, it may allow for stronger verification of microarray findings.

With the proliferation of microarray data from both in vitro and in vivo studies, it is clear that communication of this data is important to avoid replication of effort. DNA microarray data analysis has been used previously to identify marker genes or gene expression signatures which discriminate cancer from normal samples. Because studies may be limited in sample size, it may be difficult to find common markers among different studies of the same cancer type. One approach to this has been to perform cross-platform validation using a new classifier referred to as the top-scoring pair classifier.[67] The authors identified a pair of marker genes by integrating microarray data sets across three different prostate cancer studies that was robust in comparison of relative expression values. This approach could potentially increase the power of analysis, with the caution that the techniques employed between laboratories be standardized.

One of the difficulties in using gene expression signatures based on DNA microarrays has been that the number of genes used to create the signature may be unmanageably large or variable across studies as mentioned earlier. To address this, Rhodes et al[68] developed another statistical method they term comparative meta-profiling, to identify and assess the "intersection" of gene expression signatures. To do this, they collected the original data from 40 published cancer microarray data sets, made up of 38 million gene expression values from over 3700 cancer samples. They used this to characterize a common profile, transcriptionally activated in many cancer types relative to their normal tissues. This was further validated on twelve independent data sets. This meta-signature was not able to predict cancer versus normal in all data sets, but was highly suggestive of such in most of the 39 data sets analyzed.

Protein Microarrays

Protein microarray based approaches have been used in a variety of cancer cell types as well. Lung cancers are exemplary histologies amenable to the utility of this technique. This is presumptively due to the large set of markers typically seen in this heterogenic cancer. Zhong et al[69] used a T7 phage cDNA library of nonsmall cell lung cancer to select for tumor associated proteins from normal and nonsmall cell lung cancer patient plasmas. These were applied to microarray slides, and identified 212 immunogenic phage-expressed proteins from over 4000 clones using high-throughput screening. This was then assayed with 40 cancer and 41 normal patient samples, with 20 patient and 21 normal plasma samples used to determine the predictive value of each marker. Interestingly, there was antibody reactivity to 7 unique phage expressed proteins that were statistically significantly different between the patient and normal groups. Five of the most predictive proteins were combined in a model that was 90% sensitive and 95% specific in prediction of patient samples. This shows great promise when applied to large-scale screening of cancer cell types to evaluate downstream effects of transcriptional alterations.

Tissue Microarrays

One of the advantages of tissue microarrays is the ability to use archived tissue to study components of pathways not previously recognized in tumorigenesis in that cancer cell type. Kang et al[70] used this in demonstrating the importance of overexpression of Met (the hepatocyte growth factor receptor) in breast cancer tumorigenesis. Another advantage of this approach is the availability of long-term patient outcome data linked to the archival tissue samples. Sixty-one percent of patients who overexpressed the cytoplasmic tail of Met died of breast cancer within this 30 year time frame compared to 41% who had lower levels of expression in univariate analysis.

Likewise, Bubendorf et al[71] first surveyed gene amplifications during the process of prostate cancer progression, and were later able to clinically validate these candidate genes using tissue microarrays.[72]

Clinical Trials Using Microarray

Currently, there are many clinical trials that incorporate microarray in their evaluation of data. We shall present a few examples here. One preventive trial, NCT00161226, is a randomized controlled study investigating the efficacy of levonorgestrel for the prevention of endometrial cancer and will use microarray to evaluate the expression of genes in the endometrial lining in these patients. Another trial, NCT00166855, has as the central hypothesis that the angiogenesis related gene expression profiles from bone marrow in patients with multiple myeloma will correlate with bone marrow perfusion patterns imaged by dynamic MRI, and can even predict the clinical outcome of multiple myeloma. The principal investigators in this study plan to further validate these genes with real-time PCR, ELISA, and proteomic analysis to determine which novel molecules have the greatest clinical relevance. A randomized Phase II study of dose-adjusted EPOCH-Rituximab-bortezomib induction in patients with untreated mantle cell lymphoma, NCT00114738, incorporates sequential tumor biopsies for microarray analysis along with assessment of the clinical activity and biological effects of various combinations of chemotherapeutic agents. The goal here is to allow for each patient to serve as their own control, and potentially identify markers of therapy success or failure. In the study of breast cancer, one trial, NCT00083733, has as its' specific goal the analysis and comparison of genes and proteins in normal breast tissue to those in multiple tissues from women with breast cancer. This will allow for both genetic, epigenetic, and proteomic studies both in the same patient and among patients. This study has many objectives, including the definition of the molecular profile of primary and metastatic tumors, normal breast tissue in patients of many different risk profiles, and the establishment of cell lines from metastatic breast cancer to enable future research linked to the genetic expression data. Another breast cancer trial, NCT00088829, incorporates microarray to analyze the genetic basis of individual patient's response to treatment. Although these trials hold promise in uncovering some of the genetic pathways for cancer development, progression and response to treatment, almost all are purely analytic in their collection of microarray data. Using microarray-based profiling to stratify patients for treatment remains a prospect for the future.

References

1. Dean M. Cancer as a complex developmental disorder—nineteenth Cornelius P. Rhoads Memorial Award Lecture. Cancer Res 1998; 58(24):5633-5636.
2. Solomon E, Borrow J, Goddard AD. Chromosome aberrations and cancer. Science 1991; 254(5035):1153-1160.
3. Fearon ER, Vogelstein B. A genetic model for colorectal tumorigenesis. Cell 1990; 61(5):759-767.
4. Hanahan D, Weinberg RA. The hallmarks of cancer. Cell 2000; 100(1):57-70.
5. Ha PK, Benoit NE, Yochem R et al. A transcriptional progression model for head and neck cancer. Clin Cancer Res 2003; 9(8):3058-3064.
6. Dave SS, Wright G, Tan B et al. Prediction of survival in follicular lymphoma based on molecular features of tumor-infiltrating immune cells. N Engl J Med 2004; 351(21):2159-2169.
7. van de Vijver MJ, He YD, van't Veer LJ et al. A gene-expression signature as a predictor of survival in breast cancer. N Engl J Med 2002; 347(25):1999-2009.
8. Zhu H, Klemic JF, Chang S et al. Analysis of yeast protein kinases using protein chips. Nat Genet 2000; 26(3):283-289.
9. Houseman BT, Mrksich M. Carbohydrate arrays for the evaluation of protein binding and enzymatic modification. Chem Biol 2002; 9(4):443-454.
10. Kononen J, Bubendorf L, Kallionimeni A et al. Tissue microarrays for high-throughput molecular profiling of tumor specimens. 1998; 4(7):844-847, (1998/07//print).
11. Baghdoyan S, Roupioz Y, Pitaval A et al. Quantitative analysis of highly parallel transfection in cell microarrays. Nucleic Acids Res 2004; 32(9):e77.
12. Kuruvilla FG, Shamji AF, Sternson SM et al. Dissecting glucose signalling with diversity-oriented synthesis and small-molecule microarrays. Nature 2002; 416(6881):653-657.
13. Lockhart DJ, Dong H, Byrne MC et al. Expression monitoring by hybridization to high-density oligonucleotide arrays. Nat Biotechnol 1996; 14(13):1675-1680.
14. Pietu G, Alibert O, Guichard V et al. Novel gene transcripts preferentially expressed in human muscles revealed by quantitative hybridization of a high density cDNA array. Genome Res 1996; 6(6):492-503.
15. DeRisi J, Penland L, Brown PO et al. Use of a cDNA microarray to analyse gene expression patterns in human cancer. Nat Genet 1996; 14(4):457-460.
16. Perou CM, Sorlie T, Eisen MB et al. Molecular portraits of human breast tumours. Nature 2000; 406(6797):747-752.
17. van 't Veer LJ, Dai H, van de Vijver MJ et al. Gene expression profiling predicts clinical outcome of breast cancer. Nature 2002; 415(6871):530-536.
18. Ma XJ, Salunga R, Tuggle JT et al. Gene expression profiles of human breast cancer progression. Proc Natl Acad Sci USA 2003; 100(10):5974-5979.
19. Golub TR, Slonim DK, Tamayo P et al. Molecular classification of cancer: Class discovery and class prediction by gene expression monitoring. Science 1999; 286(5439):531-537.
20. Alizadeh AA, Eisen MB, Davis RE et al. Distinct types of diffuse large B-cell lymphoma identified by gene expression profiling. Nature 2000; 403(6769):503-511.
21. Templin MF, Stoll D, Schwenk JM et al. Protein microarrays: Promising tools for proteomic research. Proteomics 2003; 3(11):2155-2166.
22. MacBeath G. Protein microarrays and proteomics. Nat Genet 2002; 32(Suppl):526-532.
23. Zhu H, Bilgin M, Bangham R et al. Global analysis of protein activities using proteome chips. Science 2001; 293(5537):2101-2105.
24. Houseman BT, Huh JH, Kron SJ et al. Peptide chips for the quantitative evaluation of protein kinase activity. Nat Biotechnol 2002; 20(3):270-274.
25. Ge H. UPA, a universal protein array system for quantitative detection of protein-protein, protein-DNA, protein-RNA and protein-ligand interactions. Nucleic Acids Res 2000; 28(2):e3.

26. Liotta LA, Espina V, Mehta AI et al. Protein microarrays: Meeting analytical challenges for clinical applications. Cancer Cell 2003; 3(4):317-325.
27. Hicks DG, Tubbs RR. Assessment of the HER2 status in breast cancer by fluorescence in situ hybridization: A technical review with interpretive guidelines. Hum Pathol 2005; 36(3):250-261.
28. Wheeler DB, Bailey SN, Guertin DA et al. RNAi living-cell microarrays for loss-of-function screens in Drosophila melanogaster cells. Nat Methods 2004; 1(2):127-132.
29. Emmert-Buck MR, Bonner RF, Smith PD et al. Laser capture microdissection. Science 1996; 274(5289):998-1001.
30. Segal JP, Stallings NR, Lee CE et al. Use of laser-capture microdissection for the identification of marker genes for the ventromedial hypothalamic nucleus. J Neurosci 2005; 25(16):4181-4188.
31. Wang E, Miller LD, Ohnmacht GA et al. High-fidelity mRNA amplification for gene profiling. Nat Biotechnol 2000; 18(4):457-459.
32. Aoyagi K, Tatsuta T, Nishigaki M et al. A faithful method for PCR-mediated global mRNA amplification and its integration into microarray analysis on laser-captured cells. Biochem Biophys Res Commun 2003; 300(4):915-920.
33. Polacek DC, Passerini AG, Shi C et al. Fidelity and enhanced sensitivity of differential transcription profiles following linear amplification of nanogram amounts of endothelial mRNA. Physiol Genomics 2003; 13(2):147-156.
34. Zhao H, Hastie T, Whitfield ML et al. Optimization and evaluation of T7 based RNA linear amplification protocols for cDNA microarray analysis. BMC Genomics 2002; 3(1):31.
35. Simone NL, Bonner RF, Gillespie JW et al. Laser-capture microdissection: Opening the microscopic frontier to molecular analysis. Trends Genet 1998; 14(7):272-276.
36. Pollack JR, Perou CM, Alizadeh AA et al. Genome-wide analysis of DNA copy-number changes using cDNA microarrays. Nat Genet 1999; 23(1):41-46.
37. Zardo G, Tiirikainen MI, Hong C et al. Integrated genomic and epigenomic analyses pinpoint biallelic gene inactivation in tumors. Nat Genet 2002; 32(3):453-458.
38. Schwaenen C, Nessling M, Wessendorf S et al. Automated array-based genomic profiling in chronic lymphocytic leukemia: Development of a clinical tool and discovery of recurrent genomic alterations. Proc Natl Acad Sci USA 2004; 101(4):1039-1044.
39. Paris PL, Andaya A, Fridlyand J et al. Whole genome scanning identifies genotypes associated with recurrence and metastasis in prostate tumors. Hum Mol Genet 2004; 13(13):1303-1313.
40. Callagy G, Pharoah P, Chin SF et al. Identification and validation of prognostic markers in breast cancer with the complementary use of array-CGH and tissue microarrays. J Pathol 2005; 205(3):388-396.
41. Weiss MM, Kuipers EJ, Postma C et al. Genomic alterations in primary gastric adenocarcinomas correlate with clinicopathological characteristics and survival. Cell Oncol 2004; 26(5-6):307-317.
42. Martinez-Climent JA, Alizadeh AA, Segraves R et al. Transformation of follicular lymphoma to diffuse large cell lymphoma is associated with a heterogeneous set of DNA copy number and gene expression alterations. Blood 2003; 101(8):3109-3117.
43. The International HapMap Project. Nature 2003; 426(6968):789-796.
44. Gabriel SB, Schaffner SF, Nguyen H et al. The structure of haplotype blocks in the human genome. Science 2002; 296(5576):2225-2229.
45. Judson R, Salisbury B, Schneider J et al. How many SNPs does a genome-wide haplotype map require? Pharmacogenomics 2002; 3(3):379-391.
46. Matsuzaki H, Loi H, Dong S et al. Parallel genotyping of over 10,000 SNPs using a one-primer assay on a high-density oligonucleotide array. Genome Res 2004; 14(3):414-425.
47. Liu S, Li Y, Fu X et al. Analysis of the factors affecting the accuracy of detection for single base alterations by oligonucleotide microarray. Exp Mol Med 2005; 37(2):71-77.
48. Zhou X, Rao NP, Cole SW et al. Progress in concurrent analysis of loss of heterozygosity and comparative genomic hybridization utilizing high density single nucleotide polymorphism arrays. Cancer Genet Cytogenet 2005; 159(1):53-57.
49. Irving JA, Bloodworth L, Bown NP et al. Loss of heterozygosity in childhood acute lymphoblastic leukemia detected by genome-wide microarray single nucleotide polymorphism analysis. Cancer Res 2005; 65(8):3053-3058.
50. Evans DM, Cardon LR. Guidelines for genotyping in genomewide linkage studies: Single-nucleotide-polymorphism maps versus microsatellite maps. Am J Hum Genet 2004; 75(4):687-692.
51. Middleton FA, Pato MT, Gentile KL et al. Genomewide linkage analysis of bipolar disorder by use of a high-density single-nucleotide-polymorphism (SNP) genotyping assay: A comparison with microsatellite marker assays and finding of significant linkage to chromosome 6q22. Am J Hum Genet 2004; 74(5):886-897.

52. Nal B, Mohr E, Ferrier P. Location analysis of DNA-bound proteins at the whole-genome level: Untangling transcriptional regulatory networks. Bioessays 2001; 23(6):473-476.
53. Blais A, Dynlacht BD. Devising transcriptional regulatory networks operating during the cell cycle and differentiation using ChIP-on-chip. Chromosome Res 2005; 13(3):275-288.
54. Ren B, Robert F, Wyrick JJ et al. Genome-wide location and function of DNA binding proteins. Science 2000; 290(5500):2306-2309.
55. Orlando V. Mapping chromosomal proteins in vivo by formaldehyde-crosslinked-chromatin immunoprecipitation. Trends Biochem Sci 2000; 25(3):99-104.
56. Darville MI, Terryn S, Eizirik DL. An octamer motif is required for activation of the inducible nitric oxide synthase promoter in pancreatic beta-cells. Endocrinology 2004; 145(3):1130-1136.
57. Palmiter RD, Haines ME. Regulation of protein synthesis in chick oviduct. 4th, Role of testosterone. J Biol Chem 1973; 248(6):2107-2116.
58. Tenenbaum SA, Carson CC, Atasoy U et al. Genome-wide regulatory analysis using en masse nuclear run-ons and ribonomic profiling with autoimmune sera. Gene 2003; 317(1-2):79-87.
59. Mazzanti CM, Tandle A, Lorang D et al. Early genetic mechanisms underlying the inhibitory effects of endostatin and fumagillin on human endothelial cells. Genome Res 2004; 14(8):1585-1593.
60. Feldman AL, Stetler-Stevenson WG, Costouros NG et al. Modulation of tumor-host interactions, angiogenesis, and tumor growth by tissue inhibitor of metalloproteinase 2 via a novel mechanism. Cancer Res 2004; 64(13):4481-4486.
61. Mazzanti C, Zeiger MA, Costouros NG et al. Using gene expression profiling to differentiate benign versus malignant thyroid tumors. Cancer Res 2004; 64(8):2898-2903.
62. Rosen J, He M, Umbricht C et al. A six gene model for differentiating benign from malignant thyroid tumors based on gene expression. Surgery 2005; 138(6):1050-6.
63. Eschrich S, Yang I, Bloom G et al. Molecular staging for survival prediction of colorectal cancer patients. J Clin Oncol 2005; 23(15):3526-3535.
64. Glinsky GV, Berezovska O, Glinskii AB. Microarray analysis identifies a death-from-cancer signature predicting therapy failure in patients with multiple types of cancer. J Clin Invest 2005; 115(6):1503-1521.
65. Sanchez-Carbayo M, Socci ND, Lozano JJ et al. Gene discovery in bladder cancer progression using cDNA microarrays. Am J Pathol 2003; 163(2):505-516.
66. Kim JM, Sohn HY, Yoon SY et al. Identification of gastric cancer-related genes using a cDNA microarray containing novel expressed sequence tags expressed in gastric cancer cells. Clin Cancer Res 2005; 11(2 Pt 1):473-482.
67. Xu L, Tan AC, Naiman DQ et al. Robust prostate cancer marker genes emerge from direct integration of inter-study microarray data. Bioinformatics 2005; 21(20):3905-3911.
68. Rhodes DR, Yu J, Shanker K et al. Large-scale meta-analysis of cancer microarray data identifies common transcriptional profiles of neoplastic transformation and progression. Proc Natl Acad Sci USA 2004; 101(25):9309-9314.
69. Zhong L, Hidalgo GE, Stromberg AJ et al. Using protein microarray as a diagnostic assay for nonsmall cell lung cancer. Am J Respir Crit Care Med 2005; 172(10):1308-1314.
70. Kang JY, Dolled-Filhart M, Ocal IT et al. Tissue microarray analysis of hepatocyte growth factor/Met pathway components reveals a role for Met, matriptase, and hepatocyte growth factor activator inhibitor 1 in the progression of node-negative breast cancer. Cancer Res 2003; 63(5):1101-1105.
71. Bubendorf L, Kononen J, Koivisto P et al. Survey of gene amplifications during prostate cancer progression by high-throughout fluorescence in situ hybridization on tissue microarrays. Cancer Res 1999; 59(4):803-806.
72. Mousses S, Bubendorf L, Wagner U et al. Clinical validation of candidate genes associated with prostate cancer progression in the CWR22 model system using tissue microarrays. Cancer Res 2002; 62(5):1256-1260.

CHAPTER 11

Gene Expression Profiling in Malignant Lymphomas

Sarah E. Henrickson, Elena M. Hartmann, German Ott
and Andreas Rosenwald*

Abstract

The practice of clinical medicine and the process of biomedical research have been transformed by the decoding of the human genome. The use of DNA microarrays to find gene expression patterns in disease and biological processes has already begun to have a significant impact on modern medicine. The study of hematological malignancies has particularly benefited from gene expression profiling, including discoveries about prognosis, mechanism and efficacious choice of therapeutic regimens. DNA microarrays have led to the discovery of better prognostic tools, including the use of Zap-70 in B-Cell Chronic Lymphocytic Leukemia (B-CLL) as an indicator of worse prognosis. Studies of Diffuse Large B-cell Lymphoma (DLBCL) have defined two molecular subgroups, with significantly different mortality rates and responses to conventional therapy. In Follicular Lymphoma (FL), the variable clinical course could be associated with molecular signatures reflecting a possible interaction between tumor cells and infiltrating immune cells. The molecular mechanisms of Mantle Cell Lymphoma (MCL) have also begun to be clarified, with a more detailed understanding of the roles of cell cycle and DNA damage pathways that are responsible for the varying degree of tumor cell proliferation and different clinical outcome in this lymphoma. While important discoveries have been made in leukemias, lymphomas and many other cancer subtypes using gene expression profiling, there are many questions left to study and the translation of these tools and their results into the clinic has just begun.

Introduction

With the development of gene expression analysis at the genomic scale comes the possibility of accurately stratifying cancer patients by the molecular characteristics of their tumors and the development of individualized, tumor-specific therapy. We currently use histological examination of cancer specimens, clinical characteristics of patients and, more recently, genetic information to classify tumors into pathological entities and to stratify cancer patients into treatment paradigms. For example, the current diagnosis of follicular lymphoma (FL) brings together morphological aspects of the tumor cell infiltrate (atypical follicular structures), immunophenotyping of the tumor cells (e.g., coexpression of the markers CD10 and BCL2) and cytogenetics (translocation of the *BCL2* oncogene).[1]

Gene expression profiling provides the potential to gain a deeper understanding of the complex biological and molecular basis of lymphomas, facilitating discovery of new drug

*Corresponding Author: Andreas Rosenwald—Institute of Pathology, University of Würzburg, Würzburg, Germany. Email: Rosenwald@mail.uni-wuerzburg.de

Microarray Technology and Cancer Gene Profiling, edited by Simone Mocellin.
©2007 Landes Bioscience and Springer Science+Business Media.

targets and new therapeutic regimens. In addition, while the most basic goals of diagnosis in the clinical setting are to clarify for the patient and the care provider both a clear prognosis and a therapeutic plan, our current standard of diagnosis does not reliably yield either. Within diagnostic categories there can be great variation among patients both in their response to therapeutic regimens and their overall survival. This situation provides the opportunity for molecular diagnostics to be developed which may help to provide clear definitions of various forms of cancer, and allow more accurate diagnosis and more applicable therapy. This will hopefully lead to more effective outcome prediction for lymphoma patients, for whom there is currently considerable variation in their clinical course even within one single lymphoma entity. Currently, accurate prognostic markers for use at the time of diagnosis as well as therapeutic alternatives are lacking in many lymphomas.

While high-throughput genomic techniques are applicable to all facets of human pathology, lymphomas will be the specific focus of this chapter. The use in clinical practice is not the only goal of gene expression profiling. Careful characterization of the patterns of gene expression of cancer cells versus normal cells can clarify the cells of origin of these conditions and the pathways that are altered during neoplastic transformation. With a clearer understanding of the mechanisms of transformation of normal cells into cancerous cells, it will be possible to design more targeted therapies with greater efficacy and fewer side effects.

Gene Expression Profiling

Gene expression profiling is based on the use of DNA microarrays to assess the level of gene expression at a given time in a population of cells. There are two main forms of microarrays.[2] The first involves the use of robotic equipment to spot complementary DNAs (cDNAs) onto glass slides coated to bind DNA effectively.[3,4] The cDNAs are attached to the slides in carefully planned grids, which allows accurate analysis of sample binding patterns after experiments take place. In order to use these arrays, the cell sample of choice is lysed, mRNA is extracted and reverse transcribed to cDNA which is fluorescently labeled. These fluorescently labeled probes are allowed to anneal to the cDNA microarray and the degree of hybridization is assessed by fluorescent microscopy. An example of this type of DNA microarray is the "Lymphochip" which contains cDNAs that are thought to be involved with the initiation and pathogenesis of leukemia and lymphoma, as well as genes thought to be generally involved in immune function.[3] This platform was created before DNA microarrays were widely available commercially. The genes on the Lymphochip were chosen by sequencing cDNA from libraries of germinal center B-cells, leukemias and lymphomas, yielding 15,000 expressed sequence tags (ESTs) enriched in immune cells.[5] Approximately 3500 additional genes were added to this pool based on their known roles in immune system function.

A second type of DNA microarray is that provided by Affymetrix. This technique uses multiple representative oligonucleotides for each gene of interest which are synthesized directly onto silicon wafers. In addition, for each oligonucleotide there is a "mismatch" probe arrayed on the chip as well, with a slightly altered sequence. Samples are prepared in a similar manner as for the cDNA arrays, although there is one round of RNA amplification added in the Affymetrix protocol. Pairing of sample cDNA to the perfect match oligonucleotide alone (with no binding to the mismatch sequence) is considered evidence of gene expression in that sample.

Gene Expression Analysis

The quantity of data generated using these techniques required the development of new analytical techniques to find the patterns and alterations of relevant pathways among all the less important changes in gene expression (noise). There are two main paradigms of analysis that have emerged. The first is based on the idea that the answer should come from the data itself, without any input from the researcher, which is known as an unsupervised approach. The preferred method of analysis in this case is often hierarchical clustering.[6] This technique uses an algorithm to cluster together genes with correlated expression or samples with similar gene expression patterns (or both) simply based upon the intrinsic relationships among gene expression patterns.

An example of a different approach is the search for genes that could differentiate between predefined cancer or lymphoma subgroups, e.g., between immunoglobulin heavy chain (IgVH) -mutated and -unmutated B-cell chronic lymphocytic leukemia (B-CLL) patients (see below).[7] This method of analysis is based on the concept that the data should follow known biological principles and is generally regarded as supervised analysis.[8] In this case, a model is designed to distinguish between a chosen number of groups, rather than being allowed to discover as many groups as it finds in the data.[9] An example of unsupervised analysis is the discovery of two subgroups of diffuse large B-cell lymphomas (DLBCL), termed activated B-cell-like (ABC) and germinal center B-cell-like (GCB) DLBCL that are biologically distinct and associated with a different clinical course.[10]

Once genes are clustered, based on similarity in gene expression, we can identify gene expression signatures that represent sets of genes which all participate in a biological process or characterize a given cell type.[11,12] For example, signatures can be derived for nontransformed B and T cells, allowing the identification of novel or unrecognized genes involved in these immune cells by their coordinate expression with genes known to be expressed by these cells (i.e., TCRα, TCRβ and CD3ζ in T cells).[12]

In addition, this allows us to derive biological meaning from the genomic data by identifying relevant cell types and important pathways in the lymphoma samples. For example, in the studies of DLBCL patients, the 'proliferation signature' was found to be associated with adverse clinical outcome, whereas expression of the 'lymph node signature' which is composed of genes mostly derived from nonmalignant bystander cells in the lymphoma specimens confers a more favorable clinical course.[11] Recognition of these gene signatures allows a better understanding of the biological processes and pathways involved in a given sample, and fosters development of prognosis prediction algorithms. Representative genes from each of the prognostically informative signatures can be combined into prognostic predictors that can be used to classify patients into prognostic and therapeutic groups.

The Applications of Gene Expression Profiling to Leukemia and Lymphoma

Diffuse Large B-Cell Lymphoma (DLBCL)

Diffuse large B-cell lymphoma is the most common lymphoma in adults.[13] While many therapeutic regimens have been attempted, the previous standard of care, CHOP (an anthracycline based chemotherapeutic regimen) was able to cure DLBCL in only 35-40% of patients.[13] Attempts to improve survival with multiple alternate regimes did not make significant changes in that success rate.[14] However, the addition of Rituximab (a monoclonal anti-CD20 antibody) to the traditional CHOP regimen did lead to a significant increase in survival,[15] although prognosis for any individual patient remains challenging to predict. It was therefore hypothesized that the failure to improve DLBCL cure rates may reflect the existence of multiple subgroups of patients, each with a slightly different pathogenic mechanism. This would imply that one particular therapeutic regimen may not be equally effective among different DLBCL subgroups. A number of methods exist for stratifying DLBCL patients in order to predict outcome, including the currently used International Prognostic Index (IPI) which focuses on clinical parameters that include: Age of the patient, Eastern Cooperative Oncology Group (ECOG) performance status, tumor stage, lactate dehydrogenase level, and the number of sites of extranodal disease.[16] However, the IPI is not able to stratify patients into different therapeutic regimens effectively.

In order to determine whether or not DLBCL is a single condition, which simply required discovery of a novel therapeutic regimen, or multiple conditions each of which required different therapies, gene expression profiling was undertaken. The initial study by Alizadeh and colleagues found two groups of DLBCL patients by hierarchical clustering.[10] In this study, gene expression patterns from the patient samples were compared to gene expression patterns from normal B lymphocyte subsets, allowing parallels to be drawn between the lymphoma samples and possible cells of origin. The first patient subgroup, which was characterized by germinal center B-cell-like (GCB) gene expression patterns, had a better prognosis with CHOP-based therapy than the second group, which was characterized by activated B-cell-like (ABC) gene expression patterns. A follow-up study from the same group used a larger patient cohort and confirmed the existence of GCB- and ABC-like subsets of DLBCL. In addition, a third DLBCL subgroup (Unclassified DLBCL) was detected that did not show characteristic gene expression patterns of GCB or ABC DLBCL.[11] Importantly, these subgroups were independent of the IPI and only partially correlated with the histological diagnosis with centroblastic monomorphic cases being more common among GCB DLBCL, while centroblastic polymorphic and immunoblastic cases were more frequently observed in ABC DLBCL.

The two major DLBCL groups each have defining characteristics beyond clustering on DNA microarrays (Fig. 1). The germinal center B-cell-like designation is prognostically favorable (five year survival of 60% versus 35% for ABC DLBCL).[11] This group was also found to more commonly have Bcl-2 translocations and c-rel amplifications than ABC DLBCL.[11] Additional differences in genetic alterations include more frequent chromosomal gains of 12q in GCB DLBCL, whereas genomic gains in 3q and 18q are predominantly found in ABC DLBCL (unpublished data). In contrast, only in cell lines representing the ABC DLBCL subgroup there was constitutive NF-κB expression.[17] NF-κB is regulated by the IκB family, which retains NF-κB in the cytoplasm until IκB kinase (IKK) phosphorylates IκBs. This targets IkBs for ubiquitin mediated proteasomal degradation, thus freeing NF-κB and allowing it to translocate to the nucleus and initiate target gene transcription.[18] NF-kB is important for normal B-cell development and survival, and constitutively nuclear NF-κB has been implicated in a number of cancers. The association of constitutive NF-κB expression in the ABC subgroup of DLBCL patients is an encouraging finding, in that it provides a novel target for drug development in the DLBCL subtype with the poorest prognosis. Interestingly, PS-341 (Velcade, Bortezomib), a proteasomal inhibitor that targets NF-kB by preventing degradation of its inhibitor, IκB, has been shown to have efficacy in treating multiple myeloma and is in trials for DLBCL patients.[19]

The microarray data allowed the diagnosis of DLBCL to go far beyond simply stratifying patients into three subgroups. A molecular predictor of survival after chemotherapy for DLBCL was created based on outcome data correlation with gene expression patterns.[11] The goal of this analysis was the identification of genes correlated with outcome, based on a Cox proportional hazards model. Genes were classified into so-called gene expression signatures that had been previously defined; genes belonging to the germinal center B-cell signature, lymph node signature and MHC class II signature were associated with good outcome in DLBCL patients, while the proliferation signature was associated with poor outcome. As expected, the expression of the germinal center B-cell signature was high in the GCB DLBCL subgroup, whereas the proliferation signature was generally more highly expressed in the ABC DLBCL subgroup. At the average, the MHC class II signature was similarly expressed in all three DLBCL groups. For the development of a gene expression-based outcome predictor, 17 genes were selected which were highly variable in expression and which represented the expression level of the respective signatures. Overall, the molecular predictor was found to be independent of the IPI.

Using Affymetrix arrays, Shipp and colleagues also studied DLBCL patients and developed a gene expression outcome predictor that included, among other genes, the expression of NOR1, PDE4B and PKC-β, which are all involved in apoptotic pathways.[20] The distinction between GCB and ABC DLBCL was also evident in this data set and the DLBCL subgroups had different survival.[8] Interestingly, Shipp et al had showed in their dataset that PDE4β was overexpressed in samples from DLBCL patients with poor prognosis. They put forward a hypothesis that the resulting inhibition of cAMP would prevent apoptosis in these cells. Subsequently, PDE4β was confirmed as a target in poor prognosis DLBCLs and the apoptotic pathway blocked in DLBCL was found to be dependent on the PI3K/AKT pathway.[21]

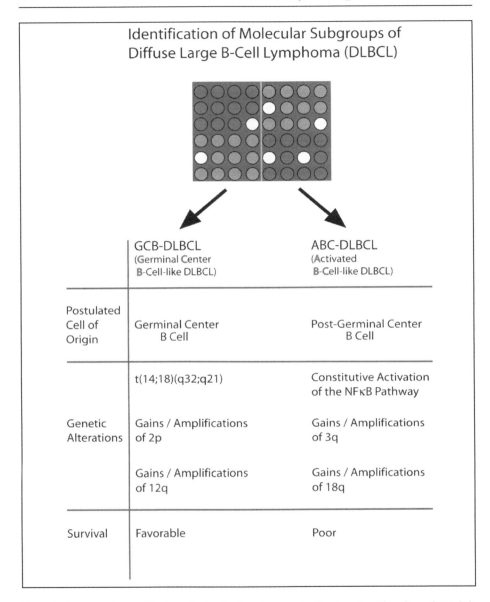

Figure 1. Gene expression profiling identified molecular subgroups of diffuse large B-cell lymphoma (DLBCL). GCB and ABC DLBCL differ in their presumed cell of origin, in underlying genetic alterations and in their clinical behavior (for details see text).

A very recent study from the same group has yielded three DLBCL subgroups by microarray profiling, with one characterized by a higher level host response, including immune cell infiltration of the tumors.[22] The importance of the tumor microenvironment in DLBCL has also recently been shown in follicular lymphoma (FL),[23] which may foreshadow more emphasis on the interaction between the lymphoma cells and the host environment in lymphoid neoplasms.

The studies by both the Shipp and Staudt groups have led to the identification of potential therapeutic targets in different subgroups of DLBCL. The Staudt group proposed the NFκB pathway as a target for ABC DLBCL.[17] The Shipp group is interested in finding inhibitors of PDE4β and the PI3K/AKT pathway as well as PKCβ, and clinical trials with a PKC-β inhibitor are ongoing (M. Shipp, personal communication).

B-Cell Chronic Lymphocytic Leukemia (B-CLL)

B-cell chronic lymphocytic leukemia (B-CLL) is the most common leukemia in the Western hemisphere.[24] However, while B-CLL is often diagnosed at an early stage of the disease, patients can either develop indolent disease or may suffer an acute, precipitous decline. Are there truly two separate types of B-CLL with separate prognostic markers and outcomes?

In order to study this question, it was necessary to find prognostic markers that identified which outcome was most likely for each patient. Initially, cytogenetic differences were studied to find prognostic markers in B-CLL, and 17p or 11q deletions were suggested to be predictors of poor outcome.[25,26]

In two independent studies, however, the presence of somatic mutations in the immuno-globulin heavy chain variable regions (IgV_H) of the tumor cells was found to be a predictor of better patient outcome.[24,27] While this finding was a landmark discovery, it is not suitable as a practical clinical test since it is expensive and time consuming to generate IgV_H sequences on all B-CLL patients, and many clinical laboratories may not have the capacity to do this test on a routine basis. In addition, it is unclear what threshold to use for differentiating IgV_H-mutated from IgV_H- unmutated B-CLL cases (thresholds from 96-98% have been used).[25] CD38 was suggested as a surrogate marker for the IgV_H mutation status; however, while CD38 expression is of prognostic significance, it failed to be confirmed as a useful surrogate marker for the IgV_H mutation status in two large studies.[25,28]

The finding of IgV_H somatic mutation levels having prognostic value might have implied that there were truly two different subtypes of B-CLL, each with their own progenitor cell, with a pregerminal B-cell in the case of IgV_H-unmutated B-CLL and a post-germinal B-cell in the case of IgV_H-mutated B-CLL. However, two separate DNA microarray studies[7,29] showed clearly that IgV_H- mutated and -unmutated B-CLLs share a homogenous gene expression signature that allows B-CLL as a whole to be distinguished from other leukemias and lymphomas. Thus, B-CLL, regardless of IgV_H somatic mutation frequency, has a distinct transcriptional profile and therefore seems to constitute one single disease.

The IgV_H mutation status therefore remained an important prognostic factor, and many groups began using the DNA microarray data to find a gene expression pattern that could serve as a proxy. While B-CLL has a generally homogenous gene expression signature across IgV_H mutated and unmutated samples, the data from gene expression studies also showed a small number of genes that had different expression levels between patients with mutated and unmutated IgV_H genes (Fig. 2).[7] The best correlate for an unmutated IgV_H status was found to be ZAP-70, a tyrosine kinase previously only known for its role in T cell receptor signaling. Interestingly, ZAP-70 was shown to be expressed at negligible levels in IgV_H mutated B-CLL cells, while it was expressed at significant levels in IgV_H unmutated B-CLL cells.[7,30,31] A large study in the UK further validated the correlation between ZAP-70 expression and the IgV_H mutation status.[32] Other groups have validated ZAP70 as a prognostic indicator as well,[33] and recently ZAP-70 has been shown to be a more useful predictor of need for therapy in B-CLL than the IgV_H mutation status.[34] In order to facilitate transfer from bench to bedside, both RT-PCR and immunohistochemical methods were developed to measure ZAP-70 levels. The use of immunohistochemistry allows proxy assessment of the IgV_H status without separating out the tumor cells, by using a concomitant stain for the B-cell marker CD19. The most promising clinical application, however, may be the measurement of ZAP-70 expression by flow cytometry analysis, since this technique is widely used in the standard work-up procedure of B-CLL samples in many laboratories.[33,34] However, many issues remain to be completely resolved, including the exact level of ZAP-70 expression necessary to be considered positive in

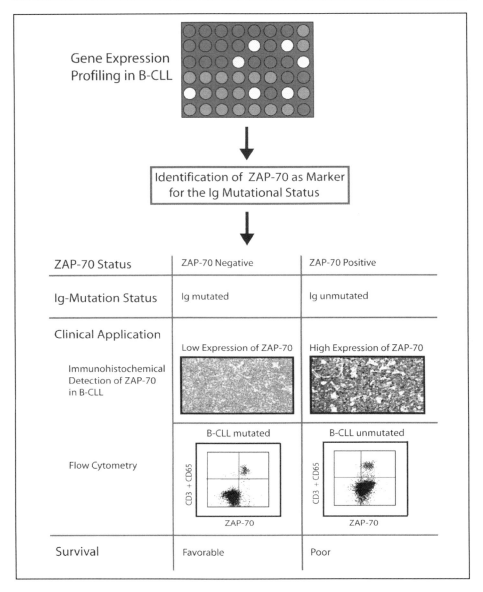

Figure 2. Gene expression profiling identified the clinical marker ZAP-70 in B-CLL. ZAP-70 appears to correlate well with the mutational status of the immunoglobulin (Ig) heavy chain gene in B-CLL cells and predicts survival of B-CLL patients. Potential applications in the routine diagnostic setting involve ZAP-70 detection by immunohistochemistry or by flow cytometry.

the various testing modalities, as well as the percentage of cells that must each be ZAP-70 positive (since there can be heterogeneity among tumor cells) and research on these issues is currently underway.

It has become clear recently that DNA damage response pathways play a role in response of B-CLL cells to therapy. There is an intriguing subset of B-CLL cases that have a shared alteration in their response to DNA damage, specifically due to ATM and p53 mutations.[35-37] As expected, with defects in DNA damage repair, these B-CLL cells have a different response to ionizing radiation than B-CLL samples with unmutated DNA damage repair genes.[38] Specifically, B-CLL cells with mutations in p53 and ATM failed to upregulate pro-apoptotic target genes (like FAS and TRAIL-receptor 2) suggesting that restoration of these mutated genes in the subset of patients with p53 and ATM mutations may have therapeutic effects.

This is especially relevant when thinking about the current therapeutic options for symptomatic B-CLL. Purine analogs, like fludarabine, act as anti-neoplastic agents by inducing double strand breaks in DNA, leading to programmed cell death. In a recent microarray study of gene expression in previously untreated B-CLL patients at 3 hours, 6 hours, and days 2, 3, 4 and 5 after initiation of fludarabine therapy, it became clear that the major alteration in gene expression was the initiation of the p53 pathway. Since there were no other clear changes in gene expression, this pathway may be the major (or exclusive) mediator of drug function.[39] This may lead to in vivo selection of p53 mutant subclones, leading to the development of drug resistant disease due to therapy. It will be important to conduct further studies on this phenomenon, including an analysis of alternate therapies and their likelihood of selecting for similar mutant B-CLL subclones.

Mantle Cell Lymphoma (MCL)

Mantle cell lymphoma (MCL) is a mature B-cell lymphoma that makes up 6% of all B-cell non-Hodgkin's lymphomas (B-NHL).[1] MCL has a median patient survival of three to four years, and while survival is heterogeneous, there is generally an aggressive clinical course with poor response to chemotherapy. The classic translocation associated with this condition is the t(11;14)(q13;q32) which leads to cyclin D1 overexpression and effects at the G1/S checkpoint of the cell cycle.[40] MCL is also associated with ATM inactivation and p53 mutations. Previous attempts to stratify MCL patients have identified characteristics associated with poor survival including a blastic morphological variant, increased tumor cell proliferation, INK4a/ARF locus deletion and p53 mutation or protein overexpression, but none of these biological features have been used to successfully stratify MCL patients into therapeutic categories.[40]

In a large gene expression profiling study, DNA microarrays of MCL patient samples were used to derive molecular prognostic information.[41] In this study, gene expression patterns of Cyclin D1-positive MCL specimens were compared to other B-NHL subsets and a large set of genes was derived that is characteristically expressed at high levels in MCL. Moreover, a small subset of MCL-like lymphoma cases were studied that show morphologic and immunophenotypic characteristics, but lack expression of Cyclin D1. A substantial proportion of these cases showed an expression profile identical to Cyclin D1-positive MCL cases and, therefore, these cases may represent a small subgroup of bona fide MCL that lack expression of Cyclin D1.

As a second step, a predictor of patient survival was constructed using the same gene expression array data. This predictor revealed that the proliferation signature was correlated with poor outcome in MCL. The predictor was optimized with a randomly selected training set of patient samples and then validated with a randomly selected validation set of patient samples. Overall, the accurate quantitative measurement of proliferation in MCL cells, provided by proliferation signature genes, identified subsets of MCL patients that differ in their survival times by almost 6 years (Fig. 3).

Several molecular features were associated with increased proliferation in MCL cells. First, higher levels of Cyclin D1 expression were found to be associated with an increase of tumor cell proliferation. MCLs can express different Cyclin D1 mRNA isoforms that differ in the lengths of their 3' untranslated regions (UTR). The 4.5kb version may have reduced stability due to a longer UTR and the presence of an RNA destabilizing element in this region. A shorter isoform of 1.7kb may be more stable due to lack of this destabilizing element. MCL cases with abundant expression of the short Cyclin D1 isoform had higher levels of overall Cyclin D1 mRNA and, therefore, an increased rate of proliferation.

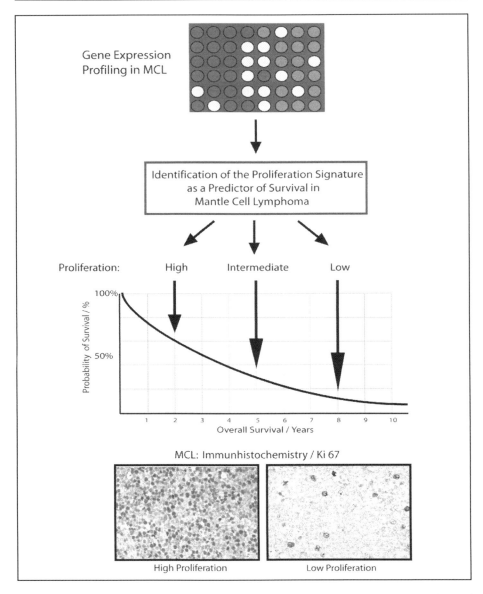

Figure 3. Gene expression profiling identified a proliferation-associated signature as a strong predictor of survival in mantle cell lymphoma (MCL). The prognosis of patients with a high score of the expression-based proliferation signature is poor, while the prognosis is more favorable in patients with a low expression of the proliferation signature. Potential clinical application involves the measurement of proliferation-associated markers by immunohistochemical methods (such as staining for Ki 67).

Second, INK4a/ARF locus deletions were found in 18/85 of the cases by quantitative PCR, and more deletions were observed among the highly proliferative cases. Interestingly, BMI-1, a transcriptional repressor of the INK4a/ARF locus was also highly expressed in a subset of highly proliferative MCL cases. In accordance with previously published data, both p53 and

ATM deletions were also found in this set of MCL patients, but neither had a strong correlation with survival or proliferation.

Interestingly, mathematical models including the level of Cyclin D1 expression or the INK4a/ARF deletion status alone or in combination did not perform as well in predicting survival than the proliferation signature-based outcome model. Thus, the gene expression-based model may capture additional oncogenic events in MCL cells that are presently not known and serve as a global integrator of molecular alterations in MCL.[41]

Follicular Lymphoma (FL)

Follicular lymphoma (FL) is the second most common form of B-cell non-Hodgkin Lymphomas (B-NHL).[1] FL is often associated with the chromosomal translocation t(14;18) that causes BCL-2 dysregulation, leading to reduced apoptosis. Clinically, there is a variable progression of the disease, from aggressive lymphoma to an indolent condition with intermittent episodes. At the present time, there are no robust biological markers available that predict the clinical course of FL patients at the time of diagnosis. In order to search for predictive markers and to identify the molecular basis of the biological and clinical heterogeneity of FL, gene expression analysis and survival signature analysis was undertaken, using RNA extracted from almost 200 FL patient samples (Fig. 4).[23] Samples were split into training and validation sets, and a statistical survival model was developed using only the training set. In particular, a Cox proportional hazards model was used to find genes associated with survival in the patient population. Hierarchical clustering was then applied to group single genes that were associated with favorable and poor survival into gene expression signatures,[12] and two of these signatures were found to have "statistical synergy": One associated with good prognosis (immune response 1) and one associated with poor prognosis (immune response 2). Interestingly, both signatures were derived from nonmalignant bystander cells in the lymph node specimens and not from the tumor cells themselves.

The signature associated with a more favorable clinical course (immune response 1) contains genes associated with subsets of T cells (e.g., CD8B1, ITK, STAT4). However, the presence of this signature is not simply due to the number of infiltrating T cells in the tumor sample, since a number of pan-T cell markers were not part of this signature. The signature associated with poor prognosis (immune response 2) contains genes associated with macrophages and dendritic cells (e.g., TLR5, LGMN and C3AR1). This model therefore predicts that the relative levels of subsets of infiltrating cells are of prognostic significance in FL, which is intriguing for understanding the pathogenesis of this condition. Future studies in FL will likely place emphasis on investigating the interaction between the neoplastic B-cells and the non-malignant bystander cells which appears to be of importance for the biological and clinical behavior of this lymphoma subtype.

A very recent study used microarray data to create a gene expression profile that could help differentiate between aggressive and indolent forms of FL, thus facilitating treatment decisions.[42] The profiles for indolent and aggressive clinical behaviour were created using sets of paired samples from indolent and aggressive stages of FL from the same patients. The final profiles allow stratification of samples into indolent and aggressive categories with a 93% success rate. This profile is not intended to project the transition from indolent to aggressive stages of the disease; it is rather a diagnostic tool to aid in therapeutic decisions. Further analysis of the genes that are more highly expressed in the aggressive form of FL may help elucidate the transition from indolent to aggressive disease.

The Future of Gene Expression Profiling in Diagnosis, Prognosis and Therapeutic Choices

Over the past six years, gene expression profiling has been used to create molecular profiles of various cancer subtypes. Lymphoid malignancies, especially the more common subtypes of B-NHL, have been well-studied and gene expression profiling data have yielded many new insights into these conditions. The first goal was to clarify whether these diseases, with historically

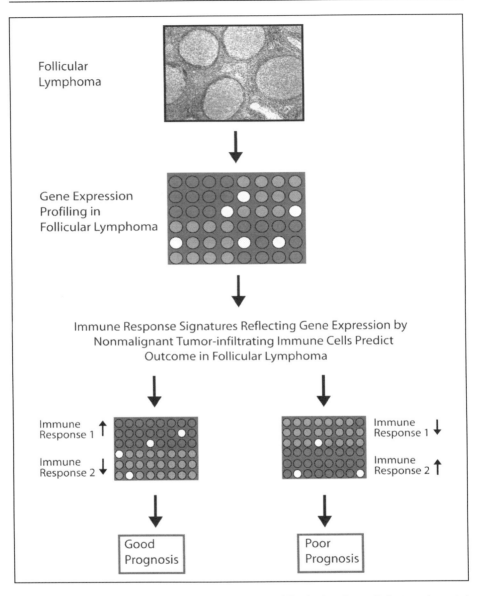

Figure 4. Immune response signatures predict outcome in follicular lymphoma (FL). A mathematical predictor using Immune Response 1 and Immune Response 2 signature genes strongly predicts outcome of FL patients at the time of diagnosis (for details see text).

diverse prognostic outcomes, are truly single conditions or diseases with multiple subgroups that might each benefit from individualized therapy. For example, the ABC and GCB-like subgroups in DLBCL represent two lymphoma subgroups with both different molecular characteristics and different responses to standard therapy. An extension of this goal is the identification of single markers for clinical/prognostic subgroups that will allow stratification of patients quickly and without the need for microarray expertise. This has been seen in B-CLL, where the identification of ZAP-70 as a proxy for the mutational status of the immunoglobulin heavy chain variable region makes the discoveries from basic science laboratories applicable to routine clinical diagnostics.

Another important goal of gene expression profiling is the identification of differentially implicated oncogenic pathways in the newly discovered subsets of lymphoid malignancies that could be targeted for future drug development. In this regard, ABC DLBCL was found to have constitutive NFκB expression and subsets of DLBCL patients are characterized by activation of PKCβ; exciting clinical trials, in which these potent oncogenic pathways are targeted by specific inhibitors, are ongoing.

It has to be noted, however, that all gene expression studies summarized in this chapter were performed in a retrospective manner, and patients had not been treated according to currently used therapeutic regimens. Thus, the benefit of molecular diagnostic studies and, in particular, of gene expression profiling, will have to be tested in future multi-center clinical trials. Once sufficient data has been collected to define molecular signatures that allow the stratification of patients into subgroups with prognostic and therapeutic implications, gene expression may make its way into the mainstream of clinical practice as an adjunct diagnostic tool. There is clearly much research left to be done both in lymphoid malignancies and beyond, but the goal is clear.

Acknowledgements

Andreas Rosenwald is supported by the Interdisciplinary Center for Clinical Research (IZKF) of the University of Würzburg, Germany. Sarah Henrickson is supported by the NIH Medical Scientist Training Program.

References

1. In: Jaffe ES, HNL Stein H, Vardiman JW, eds. World health organization classification of tumours. Pathology and Genetics of Tumours of Haematopoietic and Lymphoid Tissues. Lyon: IARC Press, 2001.
2. Staudt LM. Gene expression profiling of lymphoid malignancies. Annu Rev Med 2002; 53:303-318.
3. Alizadeh A, Eisen M, Davis RE et al. The lymphochip: A specialized cDNA microarray for the genomic-scale analysis of gene expression in normal and malignant lymphocytes. Cold Spring Harb Symp Quant Biol 1999; 64:71-78.
4. Schena M, Shalon D, Davis RW et al. Quantitative monitoring of gene expression patterns with a complementary DNA microarray. Science 1995; 270:467-470.
5. Staudt LM. Gene expression physiology and pathophysiology of the immune system. Trends Immunol 2001; 22:35-40.
6. Eisen MB, Spellman PT, Brown PO et al. Cluster analysis and display of genome-wide expression patterns. Proc Natl Acad Sci USA 1998; 95:14863-14868.
7. Rosenwald A, Alizadeh AA, Widhopf G et al. Relation of gene expression phenotype to immuno-globulin mutation genotype in B cell chronic lymphocytic leukemia. J Exp Med 2001; 194:1639-1647.
8. Wright G, Tan B, Rosenwald A et al. A gene expression-based method to diagnose clinically distinct subgroups of diffuse large B cell lymphoma. Proc Natl Acad Sci USA 2003; 100:9991-9996.
9. Braziel RM, Shipp MA, Feldman AL et al. Molecular diagnostics. Hematology (Am Soc Hematol Educ Program) 2003; 279-293.
10. Alizadeh AA, Eisen MB, Davis RE et al. Distinct types of diffuse large B-cell lymphoma identified by gene expression profiling. Nature 2000; 403:503-511.
11. Rosenwald A, Wright G, Chan WC et al. The use of molecular profiling to predict survival after chemotherapy for diffuse large-B-cell lymphoma. N Engl J Med 2002; 346:1937-1947.
12. Shaffer AL, Rosenwald A, Hurt EM et al. Signatures of the immune response. Immunity 2001; 15:375-385.
13. Coiffier B. Diffuse large cell lymphoma. Curr Opin Oncol 2001; 13:325-334.
14. Fisher RI, Gaynor ER, Dahlberg S et al. Comparison of a standard regimen (CHOP) with three intensive chemotherapy regimens for advanced nonHodgkin's lymphoma. N Engl J Med 1993; 328:1002-1006.
15. Coiffier B, Lepage E, Briere J et al. CHOP chemotherapy plus rituximab compared with CHOP alone in elderly patients with diffuse large-B-cell lymphoma. N Engl J Med 2002; 346:235-242.

16. A predictive model for aggressive nonHodgkin's lymphoma. The International NonHodgkin's Lymphoma Prognostic Factors Project. N Engl J Med 1993; 329:987-994.
17. Davis RE, Brown KD, Siebenlist U et al. Constitutive nuclear factor kappaB activity is required for survival of activated B cell-like diffuse large B cell lymphoma cells. J Exp Med 2001; 194:1861-1874.
18. Karin M, Cao Y, Greten FR et al. NF-kappaB in cancer: From innocent bystander to major culprit. Nat Rev Cancer 2002; 2:301-310.
19. Cheson BD. What is new in lymphoma? CA Cancer J Clin 2004; 54:260-272.
20. Shipp MA, Ross KN, Tamayo P et al. Diffuse large B-cell lymphoma outcome prediction by gene-expression profiling and supervised machine learning. Nat Med 2002; 8:68-74.
21. Smith PG, Wang F, Wilkinson KN et al. The phosphodiesterase PDE4B limits cAMP-associated PI3K/AKT-dependent apoptosis in diffuse large B-cell lymphoma. Blood 2005; 105:308-316.
22. Monti S, Savage KJ, Kutok JL et al. Molecular profiling of diffuse large B-cell lymphoma identifies robust subtypes including one characterized by host inflammatory response. Blood 2005; 105:1851-1861.
23. Dave SS, Wright G, Tan B et al. Prediction of survival in follicular lymphoma based on molecular features of tumor-infiltrating immune cells. N Engl J Med 2004; 351:2159-2169.
24. Damle RN, Wasil T, Fais F et al. Ig V gene mutation status and CD38 expression as novel prognostic indicators in chronic lymphocytic leukemia. Blood 1999; 94:1840-1847.
25. Krober A, Seiler T, Benner A et al. V(H) mutation status, CD38 expression level, genomic aberrations, and survival in chronic lymphocytic leukemia. Blood 2002; 100:1410-1416.
26. Dohner H, Stilgenbauer S, Benner A et al. Genomic aberrations and survival in chronic lymphocytic leukemia. N Engl J Med 2000; 343:1910-1916.
27. Hamblin TJ, Davis Z, Gardiner A et al. Unmutated Ig V(H) genes are associated with a more aggressive form of chronic lymphocytic leukemia. Blood 1999; 94:1848-1854.
28. Oscier DG, Gardiner AC, Mould SJ et al. Multivariate analysis of prognostic factors in CLL: Clinical stage, IGVH gene mutational status, and loss or mutation of the p53 gene are independent prognostic factors. Blood 2002; 100:1177-1184.
29. Klein U, Tu Y, Stolovitzky GA et al. Gene expression profiling of B cell chronic lymphocytic leukemia reveals a homogeneous phenotype related to memory B cells. J Exp Med 2001; 194:1625-1638.
30. Chen L, Apgar J, Huynh L et al. ZAP-70 directly enhances IgM signaling in chronic lymphocytic leukemia. Blood 2005; 105:2036-2041.
31. Wiestner A, Rosenwald A, Barry TS et al. ZAP-70 expression identifies a chronic lymphocytic leukemia subtype with unmutated immunoglobulin genes, inferior clinical outcome, and distinct gene expression profile. Blood 2003; 101:4944-4951.
32. Orchard JA, Ibbotson RE, Davis Z et al. ZAP-70 expression and prognosis in chronic lymphocytic leukaemia. Lancet 2004; 363:105-111.
33. Crespo M, Bosch F, Villamor N et al. ZAP-70 expression as a surrogate for immunoglobulin-variable-region mutations in chronic lymphocytic leukemia. N Engl J Med 2003; 348:1764-1775.
34. Rassenti LZ, Huynh L, Toy TL et al. ZAP-70 compared with immunoglobulin heavy-chain gene mutation status as a predictor of disease progression in chronic lymphocytic leukemia. N Engl J Med 2004; 351:893-901.
35. Stankovic T, Weber P, Stewart G et al. Inactivation of ataxia telangiectasia mutated gene in B-cell chronic lymphocytic leukaemia. Lancet 1999; 353:26-29.
36. Stankovic T, Stewart GS, Fegan C et al. Ataxia telangiectasia mutated-deficient B-cell chronic lymphocytic leukemia occurs in pregerminal center cells and results in defective damage response and unrepaired chromosome damage. Blood 2002; 99:300-309.
37. Pettitt AR, Sherrington PD, Stewart G et al. p53 dysfunction in B-cell chronic lymphocytic leukemia: Inactivation of ATM as an alternative to TP53 mutation. Blood 2001; 98:814-822.
38. Stankovic T, Hubank M, Cronin D et al. Microarray analysis reveals that TP53- and ATM-mutant B-CLLs share a defect in activating proapoptotic responses after DNA damage but are distinguished by major differences in activating prosurvival responses. Blood 2004; 103:291-300.
39. Rosenwald A, Chuang EY, Davis RE et al. Fludarabine treatment of patients with chronic lymphocytic leukemia induces a p53-dependent gene expression response. Blood 2004; 104:1428-1434.
40. Campo E, Raffeld M, Jaffe ES. Mantle-cell lymphoma. Semin Hematol 1999; 36:115-127.
41. Rosenwald A, Wright G, Wiestner A et al. The proliferation gene expression signature is a quantitative integrator of oncogenic events that predicts survival in mantle cell lymphoma. Cancer Cell 2003; 3:185-197.
42. Glas AM, Kersten MJ, Delahaye LJ et al. Gene expression profiling in follicular lymphoma to assess clinical aggressiveness and to guide the choice of treatment. Blood 2005; 105:301-307.

CHAPTER 12

Tumor Immunology

Simone Mocellin,* Mario Lise and Donato Nitti

Abstract

Advances in tumor immunology are supporting the clinical implementation of several immunological approaches to cancer in the clinical setting. However, the alternate success of current immunotherapeutic regimens underscores the fact that the molecular mechanisms underlying immune-mediated tumor rejection are still poorly understood. Given the complexity of the immune system network and the multidimensionality of tumor/host interactions, the comprehension of tumor immunology might greatly benefit from high-throughput microarray analysis, which can portrait the molecular kinetics of immune response on a genome-wide scale, thus accelerating the discovery pace and ultimately catalyzing the development of new hypotheses in cell biology. Although in its infancy, the implementation of microarray technology in tumor immunology studies has already provided investigators with novel data and intriguing new hypotheses on the molecular cascade leading to an effective immune response against cancer. Although the general principles of microarray-based gene profiling have rapidly spread in the scientific community, the need for mastering this technique to produce meaningful data and correctly interpret the enormous output of information generated by this technology is critical and represents a tremendous challenge for investigators, as outlined in the first section of this book. In the present Chapter, we report on some of the most significant results obtained with the application of DNA microarray in this oncology field.

Tumor Immunology and the Post-Genomic Era

Recent years have witnessed important breakthroughs in the understanding of tumor immunology.[1] Moreover, a variety of immunotherapeutic strategies have shown that immune manipulation can mediate the regression of established cancer in humans.[2,3] The identification of the genes encoding tumor associated antigens (TAA) and the development of therapies for immunizing against these antigens have opened new avenues for the development of an effective anticancer immunotherapy.[4] Although several immunotherapeutic approaches have demonstrated that immune cells can be polarized against tumors, in most cases the absence of correlation of these findings with clinical regression has halted back on the employment of new modalities, and cancer immunotherapy seems to have reached a plateau of results. In order to further explore the anticancer potential of the immune system, a better understanding of the finely orchestrated molecular mechanisms governing tumor/host interactions is very much needed. An efficient immune response against tumor cells comprises an intricate cross talk among cells in the tumor microenvironment. However, at present the mechanism underlying tumor immune rejection is still poorly understood. Only when the molecular matrix governing

*Corresponding Author: Simone Mocellin—Clinica Chirurgica II, Dipartimento di Scienze Oncologiche e Chirurgiche, University of Padova, Via Giustiniani 2, Padova, Italy.
Email: mocellins@hotmail.com

Microarray Technology and Cancer Gene Profiling, edited by Simone Mocellin.
©2007 Landes Bioscience and Springer Science+Business Media.

immune responsiveness of cancer is deciphered, new therapeutic strategies will be designed to fit biologically defined mechanisms of cancer immune rejection.

Traditional molecular analyses are "reductionist" as they only assess the expression of one or a few genes at a time. Thus, the output of single gene analysis is hardly applicable to biologic models whose outcome is likely to be governed by the combined influence of a global gene network. The development of other molecular methods, such as comparative genomic hybridization (CGH),[5] differential display,[6] serial analysis of gene expression (SAGE),[7] and DNA microarrays,[8] together with the sequencing of the human genome, has provided an opportunity to monitor and investigate the complex cascade of molecular events that regulate tumor-host interactions. The availability of such large amounts of information has shifted the attention of scientists from a hypothesis-driven approach to biological phenomena (the analysis of one event at a time) to a "nonreductionist" approach, where thousands of observations are recorded at once.[9] In particular, the novelty of functional genomics lies in the double opportunity to give a holistic genetic basis to hypothesis-driven approaches as well as to make unbiased observations first and then generate new, unanticipated hypotheses from those observations. Global gene-expression analysis should be of great use in the field of immunology,[10] as it has been shown clearly that the study of a single immunological parameter at one time is not sufficient to generate a general view of how the immune system fights a given pathogen or tumor, maintains self-tolerance or "memorize" past encounters with antigens.[11] The analysis of complexity in biological systems might start from a simplified representation of static gene networks moving towards an increasingly well defined and integrated description of biological phenomena, bearing in mind that only dynamic network models will probably explain reality adequately.[12]

High-throughput technologies can be used to follow changing patterns of gene expression over time. Among them, microarrays have become prominent because they are easier to use, do not require large-scale DNA sequencing, and allow the parallel quantification of thousands of genes across multiple samples.[13] Although this technology provides no information on the biologically active products of genes (i.e., proteins), functional genomics studies have demonstrated a tight correlation between the function of a protein and the expression patterns of its gene, which represents the rational for a gene profile-based formulation of scientific hypotheses.[8] However, translational gene expression regulation and post-translational protein modifications are also of crucial importance in determining cell functions. Therefore, gene microarray technology should be complemented with other recently developed high-throughput assays, such as tissue microarray[14] and proteomics.[15] Hopefully, by integrating these powerful analytic tools, investigators will be able to comprehensively describe the molecular portrait of the biological phenomena underlying tumor immune rejection.

Tumor Immune Escape

Despite the evidence that immune effectors can play a significant role in controlling tumor growth in natural conditions or in response to therapeutic manipulation, it is evident that cancer cells can survive their attack as the disease progresses. Several mechanisms underlying immune escape have been proposed, such as down-regulation of HLA molecules/TAA on tumor cell surface, the production of immunosuppressive cytokines and the expression of lymphotoxic molecules (i.e., FAS ligand) by malignant cells.[16] However, these mechanisms cannot be advocated in all cases of immunotherapy failure and some of the proposed explanations have been questioned. Therefore, other molecular events must be hypothesized in order to dissect this phenomenon that is acting as a brake for the development of effective anticancer immunotherapeutic strategies.

Gene expression profiling led investigators to hypothesize that a tumor suppressor gene (i.e., retinoic acid receptor β2, RARβ2) exerts its anticancer activity through the stimulation of the immune system.[17] RARβ2, which is inactivated in many epithelial tumors and their derived cell lines, has frequently been shown to be the principal mediator of the tumor suppressive effects of retinoic acid. Searching for genes regulated by this receptor, the authors found that several of them code for proteins favoring an effective antitumor immune response, suggesting that down-regulation of these genes in RARβ2-deficient tumor cells may contribute to immune system evasion. In this paradigmatic experience, microarray technology allowed investigators to formulate and corroborate their hypothesis by simultaneously screening several gene pathways potentially influenced by a given gene.

Several methods to make malignant cells "recognizable" by immune cells have been advocated.[18] One such method implies the exposition of target cells to sub-lethal doses of radiation. In order to dissect the molecules involved in this phenomenon of sensitization of cancer to the cytotoxic activity of the immune system, some authors utilized microarray analysis of colon, lung and prostate carcinoma cell lines treated with nonlytic doses of radiation (10-20 Gy).[19] The study allowed investigators to assess what set of genes (e.g., genes encoding TAA, adhesion molecules, cytotoxicity-related factors) are modulated in their expression by radiotherapy and may alter the phenotype of target tissue ultimately making tumor cells more susceptible to T cell-mediated immune attack. Overall, these findings might help design novel immunotherapeutic strategies able to overcome immune tolerance towards cancer.

New Targets for Tumor Immunotherapy

The molecular identification of TAA has opened new possibilities for the development of effective immunotherapies for patients with cancer. Although some TAA derive from mutated genes, most of them are products of nonmutated genes encoding intracellular proteins that are commonly expressed by autologous cancer cells.[20] Therefore, interest in antigen-specific cellular immune response has triggered enthusiasm for the development of vaccination regimens with T cell epitopes.

Classically, the identification of TAA derived T cell epitopes requires patient-derived T cells and either a gene expression approach[21] or mass spectrometry-based sequencing of the recognized peptides.[22] More recently, "reverse immunology" has been proposed as a novel approach to select HLA class I restricted epitopes from a given TAA.[23] Main drawbacks of T cell-based strategies are the time-consuming culture techniques and, more importantly, their limitation by the frequency of preexisting epitope-specific T cells. Comparative expression profiling of a tumor and the corresponding autologous normal tissue enabled by gene microarray technology is an excellent method for identifying large numbers of candidate TAA from individual tumor samples, as demonstrated by several authors.[24-28] Using this strategy, investigators have found that several genes were overexpressed by transplantable thymomas established from an inbred p53-/- mouse strain.[29] Mice were then immunized with mixtures of peptides representing putative cytotoxic T cell epitopes derived from one of the gene products identified by DNA microarray analysis. Interestingly, such immunized mice were protected against subsequent tumor challenges, showing that this gene profile based strategy is suitable for the screening of new TAA-derived immunogenic peptides. Similar findings have been already reported in humans.[30] Therefore, it seems appealing to screen the entire transcriptome of any given tumor to identify genes encoding proteins that encompass possible epitopes for peptide-based tumor-specific vaccines. A potential development of such strategy could be the utilization of microarray technology for designing patient-tailored TAA-based vaccination. To this aim, some authors have recently proposed the integration of high-density oligonucleotide array with mass spectrometry, quantitative real time PCR and HLA-tetramer technology to identify patient-specific candidate peptides suitable for anticancer vaccination.[31] After sorting out genes selectively expressed or overexpressed in malignant tissues (renal cell carcinomas), these investigators identified HLA class I-restricted peptides from tumor specimens by means of mass spectrometry. Then, peripheral CD8+ T cells from tumor patients and healthy individuals were tested for reactivity towards the candidate peptides using quantitative real time PCR and HLA-tetramer based flow cytometry, thus allowing to identify TAA epitopes potentially suitable for clinical implementation.

Dendritic Cell Biology

Although tumor cells express TAA that can be recognized by T cells, advanced tumors are generally not immunogenic, at least in part because they do not express costimulatory molecules. The fate of TAA largely depends on their ability to be phagocytosed and processed by dendritic cells, the most powerful antigen presenting cells.[32] Dendritic cells expressing high levels of HLA class I and II and costimulatory molecules have demonstrated high efficiency and potency in presenting TAA peptides to enhance cellular immunity both in preclinical models and in humans.[2,3]

Despite the strong preclinical evidence supporting the use of dendritic cells for anticancer vaccination in humans, the results of clinical trials so far carried out do not seem to meet the expectations,[2,3] likely because the physiology of these cells is only partially understood and their therapeutic potential incompletely exploited. Immature dendritic cells capture TAA in the peripheral tissues, process them into peptides bound to HLA molecules, and then migrate to lymphoid organs where they present HLA-peptide complexes to T lymphocytes. Following the interaction with TAA-specific T helper lymphocytes, dendritic cells become activated through the CD40 signaling pathway, up-regulate HLA and costimulatory molecules expression on their surface and acquire a mature phenotype, characterized by the expression of new markers such as CD83 and by the secretion of pro-inflammatory and chemotactic cytokines.[33] Gene profiling studies have recently broadened the spectrum of genes distinguishing immature versus mature dendritic cells.[34] Mature dendritic cells prime cytotoxic T lymphocytes, thus polarizing the effector arm of the cell mediated immune response against the pathogen agent. By contrast, dendritic cells conditioned by regulatory T suppressor cells are "licensed" to inhibit the initiation of the immune response by inducing T helper lymphocyte anergy. To characterize the molecular changes occurring in tolerogenic dendritic cells, some investigators investigated the mRNA profile of dendritic cells exposed to allospecific T helper and T suppressor cells, showing that immature dendritic cells conditioned by T suppressor cells differentiate into tolerogenic dendritic cells with a distinct phenotype as compared to mature nontolerogenic dendritic cells.[35] The identification of dendritic cell gene pathways induced by suppressor lymphocytes could be of paramount importance to dissect the molecular mechanisms underlying immune tolerance towards tumors and consequently to identify new strategies to circumvent this obstacle.

Yet, using DNA microarray technology, other authors described the molecular portrait characterizing dendritic cells at different stages of maturation.[36] In an animal model, these researchers could link two different dendritic cell gene patterns with two levels of effectiveness in inducing tumor regression mediated by dendritic cell-based vaccine. If confirmed in a human model, these results might explain some vaccination failures observed in the clinical setting and indicate new avenues of research in the design of more effective dendritic cell preparation protocols for antitumor vaccines. Currently, most clinical protocols imply the expansion of dendritic cells with granulocyte/monocyte colony-stimulating factor (GM-CSF) combined with interleukin-4 (IL-4), while their maturation is induced with tumor necrosis factor (TNF).[37] The microarray-based study of the cascade of molecular events leading to a successful expansion/maturation of dendritic cells has already begun,[38] and novel strategies for improving dendritic cell-based anticancer immunotherapy are expected in the near future.

T Cell Biology

As a direct consequence of TAA presentation by antigen presenting cells, naïve T cells become activated helper and cytotoxic T lymphocytes. Immune polarization can also differentially affect T cells, as demonstrated by the fact that human type 1/type 2 helper lymphocytes and cytotoxic T cell clones express substantially distinct sets of genes. In animal models it has been demonstrated that the activated tumor-specific effector T cells mainly comprise type 1 CD4+ and CD8+ lymphocytes, both of which are important for an effective antitumor immune response.[39] Thus, the cellular and molecular biology of these T cell subsets is of substantial interest in the context of both basic and clinical tumor immunology. Using microarray technology, investigators have started exploring the mRNA steady state of such tumor specific T cells as compared to naïve T cells in mice.[40] Gene expression profiling has been also applied to the study the mechanisms of partial T cell activation, which accounts for different cytotoxic capabilities and might determine the clinical outcome of vaccinated cancer bearing patients.[41] To mimic a sub-optimal cytotoxic T lymphocyte activation, investigators developed a model of naive CD8[+] T cells from transgenic mice expressing an alloreactive T cell receptor (TCR) for which a mutant alloantigen behaved as a partial agonist, inducing only some of the effector functions induced by the native alloantigen.[42] To ascertain the molecular bases for the establishment of divergent fates within the same naive CD8[+] T cells, they used cDNA microarrays to monitor sequential gene expression patterns in conditions of full or partial response of these naive CD8[+] T cells. Clusters of genes encoding costimulatory molecules and genes controlling cytolytic function, cytokine production, and chemokines were found to discriminate between partially and fully activated lymphocytes, providing new insights on the gene pathway leading to an effective immune response against cancer.

Tumor Microenvironment

Until recently, most studies addressing the immunological effects of vaccination in cancer patients have looked at variations in the level of TAA-specific reactivity in circulating lymphocytes.[43] Results from clinical trials have shown that vaccination can be quite effective in inducing tumor-specific T cell responses that can be easily observed among circulating lymphocytes.[2,3] However, the identification of such immune responses could not be consistently correlated with tumor regression. Moreover, approaching immune follow-up of vaccinated cancer patients at systemic level presents some intrinsic limitations. For instance, none of the assays currently in use can be considered ideal to reveal the activation status of anticancer immunity. Moreover, the study of circulating T cell responses yields only one type of information, though important, which consists of the documentation of whether a most often locally administered immunogen may induce a systemic effect beyond the draining lymph nodes. It is questionable, however, whether the immunogenic wave induced systemically by the vaccine reaches the tumor microenvironment. Thus, complementing the analysis of immune responses in circulating lymphocytes with the study of the tumor microenvironment may yield information about the quality and intensity of the elicited immune response within the relevant arena. To this aim, it was proposed that a dynamic analysis of host/tumor interactions following immunotherapy could be most fruitfully performed by correlating clinical outcome with the gene expression kinetics of a given tumor lesion that could be easily accessed by repeated fine needle aspirates, such as in transit melanoma metastases.[44] The application of such a strategy combined with microarray-based gene profiling led to find that melanoma metastases undergoing complete regression in response to peptide/interleukin-2 (IL-2) based vaccination were characterized by a different transcript signature as compared to those progressing.[45] Interestingly, many genes over-expressed in responding melanoma metastases were immune-related. Among them, the authors focused on TIA-1 and interleukin-10 (IL-10).[46] TIA-1 codes for a 15 kd cytotoxicity-related protein expressed by cytotoxic T lymphocytes and natural killer (NK) cells, and is characterized by pro-apoptotic properties. IL-10 is generally considered an immunosuppressive molecule that can anergize cytotoxic T lymphocytes, acting both directly and through its inhibitory effects on dendritic cells. However, several preclinical models have shown that IL-10 can also mediate tumor regression by stimulating NK cells activity.[46] Furthermore, using cDNA microarray it was observed that, in vitro, IL-10 induced NK cell (but not cytotoxic T lymphocytes) expression of cytotoxicity related genes, including TIA-1.[47] These observations led to hypothesize that, in the presence of high levels of IL-10 in the tumor microenvironment, NK cells might be stimulated to lyse cancer cells, thus increasing TAA availability and "danger signals" delivery required by dendritic cells to be activated and effectively prime cytotoxic T cells against TAA (Fig. 1). These findings support the recently

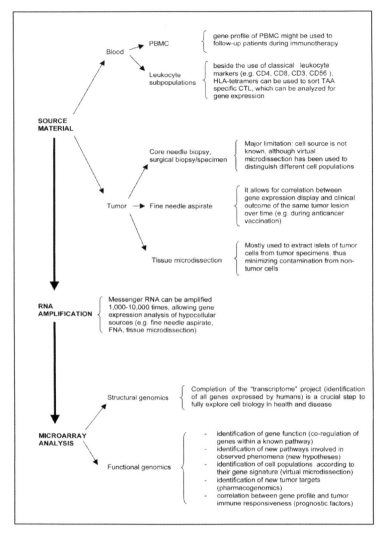

Figure 1. Example of microarray-generated hypothesis in tumor immunology. For an effective anticancer immune response to take place, a coordinated cascade of timely events are necessary. Microarray-based gene profiling of melanoma metastases in patients undergoing active specific immunotherapy showed that immune-related genes were up-regulated in responding rather than in nonresponding lesions. Among them, IL-10 and TIA-1 appeared of particular interest. In fact, IL-10 can stimulate NK cell cytotoxicity both directly (e.g., by increasing TIA-1 expression) and by decreasing macrophage production of reactive oxygen species (ROS), which are well known NK cell inhibitors. By enhancing NK cell activity, IL-10 might contribute to an effective early stage immune response because the increased tumor cell lysis offers a greater availability of TAA for dendritic cells. In addition, an increased tumor destruction amplifies the and chemotactic and danger signals, (e.g., chemotactic peptides, heat shock proteins and double stranded DNA), necessary to recruit and subsequently activate innate immunity cells and immature dendritic cells. Through the inhibition of dendritic cell maturation, IL-10 prolongs their capability for antigen uptake while simultaneously postponing their migration to draining lymph nodes until an appropriate antigen loading has occurred.

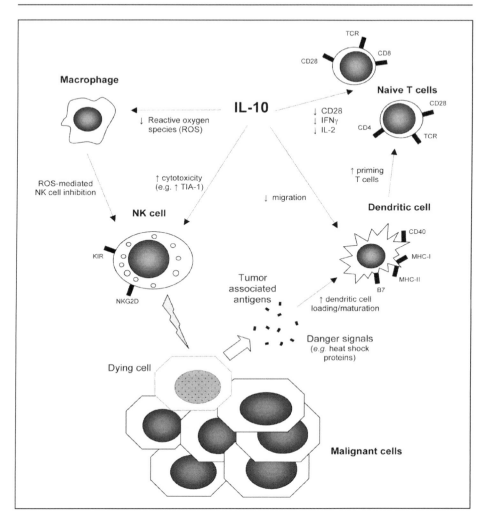

Figure 2. Global view of potential strategies and objectives for microarray-based tumor immunology studies. PBMC: peripheral blood mononuclear cells.

renewed interest in the pivotal role that NK cells may play in the early phase of adaptive immunity engagement against a noxious agent (e.g., infectious agent, tumor cells), thus providing a key link between innate and adaptive immunity.[48] If this theory were proved to be correct, future anticancer immunotherapy strategies should address the challenging task of stimulating both innate and adaptive immunity in a timely fashion.[49]

As systemic IL-2 administration significantly increases the frequency of tumor regression induced by peptide-based vaccination of melanoma patients,[50] some authors investigated the role of this cytokine in facilitating an effective immune response. It was postulated that the anticancer effects of IL-2 are mediated through in vivo expansion and activation of cytotoxic lymphocytes and/or promotion of their migration within target tissues, but it has become apparent that IL-2 at the doses used therapeutically has broader immune/pro-inflammatory effects. Which of these effects has a critical role in mediating tumor regression remains enigmatic.

In a study, early changes in transcriptional profiles of circulating mononuclear cells were compared with those occurring within the microenvironment of melanoma metastases following systemic IL-2 administration.[51] The results of this microarray-based work suggested that IL-2 administration induces three predominant effects: (a) activation of antigen-presenting monocytes; (b) a massive production of chemoattractants that may recruit other immune cells to the tumor site, among which are the chemokines MIG and PARC specific for T cells; and (c) the activation of lytic mechanisms ascribable to monocytes (calgranulin, grancalcin) and NK cells (for example, NKG5, NK4). These findings suggest that systemic IL-2 administration may facilitate T cell effector function in the target organ not by sustaining their proliferation, as generally believed, but rather by promoting their migration and by providing a milieu conducive to their activation in situ through activation of antigen-presenting cells. If this hypothesis were correct, then adoptive transfer of effector T cells should follow, rather than precede, administration of systemic IL-2.

Concluding Remarks

Although we are only beginning to exploit the enormous potential of high-throughput technologies for dissecting the molecular events governing tumor immune rejection, preliminary results prompt investigators to pursue the genomic approach to tumor immunology. In fact, the high complexity of the immune network makes difficult to understand the finely orchestrated molecular and cellular phenomena underlying tumor/host immune system interactions look-ing at the expression of one or few molecules at a time, as the traditional research approach has so far sustained. Hopefully, a global view of the expression profiles of the several key players involved in tumor immune surveillance/tolerance will enable investigators to describe the sequence of events conducive to an effective immune recognition and killing of malignant cells, thus giving the opportunity to reproduce them in a larger series of patients. Besides shedding new light on the mechanisms of cancer immune rejection, microarray technology is expected to provide investigators with other information (Fig. 2). For instance, clinicians might use gene profiling as a powerful tool to assess the activation status of the immune system (both in the peripheral blood and in the tumor microenvironment) of each patient before and during immunotherapy, thus opening the avenue to the personalization of the treatment. Only the broad implementation of microarray-generated data in the clinical protocols of anticancer immunotherapy will allow to test the theoretically invaluable potential of such an approach.

References

1. Pardoll DM. Spinning molecular immunology into successful immunotherapy. Nat Rev Immunol 2002; 2:227-38.
2. Mocellin S, Mandruzzato S, Bronte V et al. Part I: Vaccines for solid tumours. Lancet Oncol 2004; 5:681-9.
3. Mocellin S, Semenzato G, Mandruzzato S et al. Part II: Vaccines for haematological malignant disorders. Lancet Oncol 2004; 5:727-37.
4. Rosenberg SA. Progress in human tumour immunology and immunotherapy. Nature 2001; 411:380-4.
5. Pinkel D, Segraves R, Sudar D et al. High resolution analysis of DNA copy number variation using comparative genomic hybridization to microarrays. Nat Genet 1998; 20:207-11.
6. Broude NE. Differential display in the time of microarrays. Expert Rev Mol Diagn 2002; 2:209-16.
7. Velculescu VE, Zhang L, Vogelstein B et al. Serial analysis of gene expression. Science 1995; 270:484-7.
8. Brown PO, Botstein D. Exploring the new world of the genome with DNA microarrays. Nat Genet 1999; 21:33-7.
9. Goldenfeld N, Kadanoff LP. Simple lessons from complexity. Science 1999; 284:87-9.
10. Staudt LM, Brown PO. Genomic views of the immune system*. Annu Rev Immunol 2000; 18:829-59.
11. Ricciardi-Castagnoli P, Granucci F. Opinion: Interpretation of the complexity of innate immune responses by functional genomics. Nat Rev Immunol 2002; 2:881-9.
12. Keil D, Luebke RW, Pruett SB. Quantifying the relationship between multiple immunological parameters and host resistance: Probing the limits of reductionism. J Immunol 2001; 167:4543-52.

13. Mocellin S, Provenzano M, Rossi CR et al. DNA array-based gene profiling: From surgical specimen to the molecular portrait of cancer. Ann Surg 2005; 241:16-26.
14. Kallioniemi OP, Wagner U, Kononen J et al. Tissue microarray technology for high-throughput molecular profiling of cancer. Hum Mol Genet 2001; 10:657-62.
15. Le Naour F. Contribution of proteomics to tumor immunology. Proteomics 2001; 1:1295-1302.
16. Marincola FM, Jaffee EM, Hicklin DJ et al. Escape of human solid tumors from T-cell recognition: Molecular mechanisms and functional significance. Adv Immunol 2000; 74:181-273.
17. Toulouse A, Loubeau M, Morin J et al. RARbeta involvement in enhancement of lung tumor cell immunogenicity revealed by array analysis. FASEB J 2000; 14:1224-32.
18. Mocellin S, Rossi CR, Nitti D. Cancer vaccine development: On the way to break immune tolerance to malignant cells. Exp Cell Res 2004; 299:267-78.
19. Garnett CT, Palena C, Chakraborty M et al. Sublethal irradiation of human tumor cells modulates phenotype resulting in enhanced killing by cytotoxic T lymphocytes. Cancer Res 2004; 64:7985-94.
20. Renkvist N, Castelli C, Robbins PF et al. A listing of human tumor antigens recognized by T cells. Cancer Immunol Immunother 2001; 50:3-15.
21. van der Bruggen P, Traversari C, Chomez P et al. A gene encoding an antigen recognized by cytolytic T lymphocytes on a human melanoma. Science 1991; 254:1643-7.
22. Cox AL, Skipper J, Chen Y et al. Identification of a peptide recognized by five melanoma-specific human cytotoxic T cell lines. Science 1994; 264:716-9.
23. Maecker B, von B-B, Anderson KS et al. Linking genomics to immunotherapy by reverse immunology—'immunomics' in the new millennium. Curr Mol Med 2001; 1:609-19.
24. Young AN, Amin MB, Moreno CS et al. Expression profiling of renal epithelial neoplasms: A method for tumor classification and discovery of diagnostic molecular markers. Am J Pathol 2001; 158:1639-51.
25. Takahashi M, Rhodes DR, Furge KA et al. Gene expression profiling of clear cell renal cell carcinoma: Gene identification and prognostic classification. Proc Natl Acad Sci USA 2001; 98:9754-9.
26. Boer JM, Huber WK, Sultmann H et al. Identification and classification of differentially expressed genes in renal cell carcinoma by expression profiling on a global human 31,500- element cDNA array. Genome Res 2001; 11:1861-70.
27. Shi YY, Wang HC, Yin YH et al. Identification and analysis of tumour-associated antigens in hepatocellular carcinoma. Br J Cancer 2005; 92:929-34.
28. Yoshitake Y, Nakatsura T, Monji M et al. Proliferation potential-related protein, an ideal esophageal cancer antigen for immunotherapy, identified using complementary DNA microarray analysis. Clin Cancer Res 2004; 10:6437-48.
29. Mathiassen S, Lauemoller SL, Ruhwald M et al. Tumor-associated antigens identified by mRNA expression profiling induce protective anti-tumor immunity. Eur J Immunol 2001; 31:1239-46.
30. Wang T, Fan L, Watanabe Y et al. L552S, an alternatively spliced isoform of XAGE-1, is over-expressed in lung adenocarcinoma. Oncogene 2001; 20:7699-709.
31. Weinschenk T, Gouttefangeas C, Schirle M et al. Integrated functional genomics approach for the design of patient- individual antitumor vaccines. Cancer Res 2002; 62:5818-27.
32. Banchereau J, Briere F, Caux C et al. Immunobiology of dendritic cells. Annu Rev Immunol 2000; 18:767-811.
33. Lanzavecchia A, Sallusto F. Regulation of T cell immunity by dendritic cells. Cell 2001; 106:263-266.
34. Chen Z, Gordon JR, Zhang X et al. Analysis of the gene expression profiles of immature versus mature bone marrow-derived dendritic cells using DNA arrays. Biochem Biophys Res Commun 2002; 290:66-72.
35. Suciu-Foca Cortesini N, Piazza F, Ho E et al. Distinct mRNA microarray profiles of tolerogenic dendritic cells. Hum Immunol 2001; 62:1065-72.
36. Chen Z, Dehm S, Bonham K et al. DNA array and biological characterization of the impact of the maturation status of mouse dendritic cells on their phenotype and antitumor vaccination efficacy. Cell Immunol 2001; 214:60-71.
37. Figdor CG, De Vries IJ, Lesterhuis WJ et al. Dendritic cell immunotherapy: Mapping the way. Nat Med 2004; 10:475-80.
38. Ju XS, Hacker C, Madruga J et al. Towards determining the differentiation program of antigen-presenting dendritic cells by transcriptional profiling. Eur J Cell Biol 2003; 82:75-86.
39. Huang H, Li F, Gordon JR et al. Synergistic enhancement of antitumor immunity with adoptively transferred tumor-specific CD4+ and CD8+ T cells and intratumoral lymphotactin transgene expression. Cancer Res 2002; 62:2043-51.
40. Zhang X, Chen Z, Huang H et al. DNA microarray analysis of the gene expression profiles of naive versus activated tumor-specific T cells. Life Sci 2002; 71:3005-17.

41. Carrabba MG, Castelli C, Maeurer MJ et al. Suboptimal activation of CD8(+) T cells by melanoma-derived altered peptide ligands: Role of Melan-A/MART-1 optimized analogues. Cancer Res 2003; 63:1560-7.
42. Verdeil G, Puthier D, Nguyen C et al. Gene profiling approach to establish the molecular bases for partial versus full activation of naive CD8 T lymphocytes. Ann NY Acad Sci 2002; 975:68-76.
43. Keilholz U, Weber J, Finke JH et al. Immunologic monitoring of cancer vaccine therapy: Results of a workshop sponsored by the Society for Biological Therapy. J Immunother 2002; 25:97-138.
44. Wang E, Marincola FM. A natural history of melanoma: Serial gene expression analysis. Immunol Today 2000; 21:619-23.
45. Wang E, Miller LD, Ohnmacht GA et al. Prospective molecular profiling of melanoma metastases suggests classifiers of immune responsiveness. Cancer Res 2002; 62:3581-6.
46. Mocellin S, Panelli MC, Wang E et al. The dual role of IL-10. Trends Immunol 2003; 24:36-43.
47. Mocellin S, Panelli M, Wang E et al. IL-10 stimulatory effects on human NK cells explored by gene profile analysis. Genes Immun 2004; 5:621-30.
48. Kelly JM, Darcy PK, Markby JL et al. Induction of tumor-specific T cell memory by NK cell-mediated tumor rejection. Nat Immunol 2002; 3:83-90.
49. Mocellin S, Rossi C, Nitti D et al. Dissecting tumor responsiveness to immunotherapy: The experience of peptide-based melanoma vaccines. Biochim Biophys Acta Rev Cancer 2003; 1653:61-71.
50. Rosenberg SA, Yang JC, Schwartzentruber DJ et al. Immunologic and therapeutic evaluation of a synthetic peptide vaccine for the treatment of patients with metastatic melanoma. Nat Med 1998; 4:321-7.
51. Panelli MC, Wang E, Phan G et al. Gene-expression profiling of the response of peripheral blood mononuclear cells and melanoma metastases to systemic IL-2 administration. Genome Biol 2002; 3:RESEARCH0035.

Index